武汉大学
优秀博士学位论文文库
编委会

主 任 李晓红

副主任 韩 进　舒红兵　李 斐

委 员（按姓氏笔画为序）

　　　　　马费成　邓大松　边 专　刘正猷　刘耀林
　　　　　杜青钢　李义天　李建成　何光存　陈 化
　　　　　陈传夫　陈柏超　冻国栋　易 帆　罗以澄
　　　　　周 翔　周叶中　周创兵　顾海良　徐礼华
　　　　　郭齐勇　郭德银　黄从新　龚健雅　谢丹阳

武汉大学优秀博士学位论文文库

心房颤动的自主神经机制研究

Autonomic Mechanism for Atrial Fibrillation

鲁志兵 著

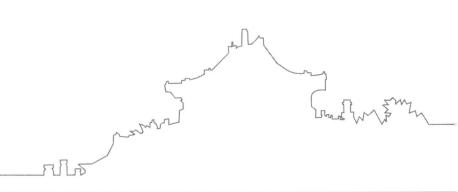

武汉大学出版社

图书在版编目(CIP)数据

心房颤动的自主神经机制研究/鲁志兵著. —武汉:武汉大学出版社,2014.1
武汉大学优秀博士学位论文文库
ISBN 978-7-307-12487-5

Ⅰ.心… Ⅱ.鲁… Ⅲ.心房纤颤—自主神经系统—研究 Ⅳ.R541.7

中国版本图书馆 CIP 数据核字(2013)第 313241 号

责任编辑:黄汉平　　责任校对:汪欣怡　　版式设计:马　佳

出版发行:武汉大学出版社　(430072　武昌　珞珈山)
　　　　　(电子邮件:cbs22@whu.edu.cn　网址:www.wdp.com.cn)
印刷:湖北恒泰印务有限公司
开本:720×1000　1/16　印张:7.5　字数:102 千字　插页:2
版次:2014 年 1 月第 1 版　2014 年 1 月第 1 次印刷
ISBN 978-7-307-12487-5　　定价:19.00 元

版权所有,不得翻印;凡购我社的图书,如有质量问题,请与当地图书销售部门联系调换。

总　　序

　　创新是一个民族进步的灵魂，也是中国未来发展的核心驱动力。研究生教育作为教育的最高层次，在培养创新人才中具有决定意义，是国家核心竞争力的重要支撑，是提升国家软实力的重要依托，也是国家综合国力和科学文化水平的重要标志。

　　武汉大学是一所崇尚学术、自由探索、追求卓越的大学。美丽的珞珈山水不仅可以诗意栖居，更可以陶冶性情、激发灵感。更为重要的是，这里名师荟萃、英才云集，一批又一批优秀学人在这里砥砺学术、传播真理、探索新知。一流的教育资源，先进的教育制度，为优秀博士学位论文的产生提供了肥沃的土壤和适宜的气候条件。

　　致力于建设高水平的研究型大学，武汉大学素来重视研究生培养，是我国首批成立有研究生院的大学之一，不仅为国家培育了一大批高层次拔尖创新人才，而且产出了一大批高水平科研成果。近年来，学校明确将"质量是生命线"和"创新是主旋律"作为指导研究生教育工作的基本方针，在稳定研究生教育规模的同时，不断推进和深化研究生教育教学改革，使学校的研究生教育质量和知名度不断提升。

　　博士研究生教育位于研究生教育的最顶端，博士研究生也是学校科学研究的重要力量。一大批优秀博士研究生，在他们学术创作最激情的时期，来到珞珈山下、东湖之滨。珞珈山的浑厚，奠定了他们学术研究的坚实基础；东湖水的灵动，激发了他们学术创新的无限灵感。在每一篇优秀博士学位论文的背后，都有博士研究生们刻苦钻研的身影，更有他们的导师的辛勤汗水。年轻的学者们，犹如在海边拾贝，面对知识与真理的浩瀚海洋，他们在导师的循循善诱下，细心找寻着、收集着一片片靓丽的贝壳，最终把它们连成一串串闪闪夺目的项链。阳光下的汗水，是他们砥砺创新的注脚；面向太阳的远方，是他们奔跑的方向；导师们的悉心指点，则是他们最值得依赖的臂膀！

　　博士学位论文是博士生学习活动和研究工作的主要成果，也是学校研究生教育质量的凝结，具有很强的学术性、创造性、规范性和专业性。博士学位论文是一个学者特别是年轻学者踏进学术之门的标志，很多博士学位论文开辟了学术领域的新思想、新观念、新视阈和新境界。

　　据统计，近几年我校博士研究生所发表的高质量论文占全校高水平论文的一半以上。至今，武汉大学已经培育出18篇"全国百篇优秀博士学位论文"，还有数十篇论文获"全国百篇优秀博士学位论文提名奖"，数百篇论文被评为"湖北省优秀博士学位论文"。优秀博士结出的累累硕果，无疑应该为我们好好珍藏，装入思想的宝库，供后学者慢慢汲取其养分，吸收其精华。编辑出版优秀博士学位论文文库，即是这一工作的具体表现。这项工作既是一种文化积累，又能助推这批青年学者更快地成长，更可以为后来者提供一种可资借鉴的范式亦或努力的方向，以鼓励他们勤于学习，善于思考，勇于创新，争取产生数量更多、创新性更强的博士学位论文。

　　武汉大学即将迎来双甲华诞，学校编辑出版该文库，不仅仅是为百廿武大增光添彩，更重要的是，当岁月无声地滑过120个春秋，当我们正大踏步地迈向前方时，我们有必要回首来时的路，我们有必要清晰地审视我们走过的每一个脚印。因为，铭记过去，才能开拓未来。武汉大学深厚的历史底蕴，不仅仅在于珞珈山的一草一木，也不仅仅在于屋檐上那一片片琉璃瓦，更在于珞珈山下的每一位学者和学生。而本文库收录的每一篇优秀博士学位论文，无疑又给珞珈山注入了新鲜的活力。不知不觉地，你看那珞珈山上的树木，仿佛又茂盛了许多！

李晓红

2013年10月于武昌珞珈山

摘 要

临床研究发现，大多数阵发性心房颤动（房颤）由肺静脉或上腔静脉内局灶快速电激动（rapid firing）诱发和驱动。应用射频能量隔离肺静脉和上腔静脉可以减少或消除房颤的发作。基础研究试图从组织学和电生理学方面探讨起源于肺静脉或上腔静脉的 rapid firing 的发生机制，但未得出一致结论。有学者认为隔离肺静脉并非根治房颤所必需，因为以心房碎裂电位（complex fractionated atrial electrograms，CFAE）或自主神经节（ganglionated plexus，GP）为靶点的导管消融术式虽然残留肺静脉电位，但同样能消除房颤。探讨 rapid firing、CFAE 和 GP 三者在房颤发生机制中的作用对于确定房颤消融术的最佳靶点十分重要。我们以前的报道揭示以 GP 为核心的心脏内在自主神经系统参与了房颤的发生机制，临床资料也提示 GP 消融可以抑制某些阵发性房颤甚至心房存在严重电重构的慢性房颤。本研究中，我们探讨 rapid firing、CFAE 和心房电重构与心脏内在自主神经系统的关系。

目的：1. 探讨肺静脉和心房起源的 rapid firing 的自主神经机制；

2. 探讨上腔静脉起源的 rapid firing 的自主神经机制；

3. 探讨 CFAE 的自主神经机制；

4. 探讨心房电重构的自主神经机制。

方法：正常成年杂种犬，分别经左右侧第四肋间开胸，暴露心脏，分离双侧迷走交感干。将多极电生理导管分别缝于左右侧肺静脉、心房和心耳，将环状电极导管经颈静脉送入上腔静脉，实验过程中记录所有电生理信号。

1. 在基础起搏条件下，依次在各部位心肌不应期内发放高频刺激诱发 rapid firing，测量诱发房颤所需最低电压（房颤阈值）。在消融同侧或对侧 GP 或静脉推注自主神经阻滞剂后观察房颤阈值的变化。

2. 观察刺激和消融"第三脂肪垫"（SVC-Ao GP）对所有部位有效不应期（ERP）和心房易颤窗口（WOV）的影响。在上腔静脉肌袖不应期内发放高频刺激诱发 rapid firing，观察消融 SVC-Ao GP 或心房表面 GP 对 rapid firing 诱发性的影响。

3. 分别在左右心耳表面应用少量乙酰胆碱（Ach）或左右侧含 GP 的脂肪垫内注射少量 Ach，观察并分析房颤发生时碎裂电位的分布及程度。消融同侧 GP 后，观察碎裂电位的变化。

4. GP 消融之前或之后，在左心耳进行快速起搏（1200bpm）并持续 6h，观察每小时各部位 ERP 和 WOV 的变化。

结果：1. rapid firing 介导的房颤能通过刺激自主神经末梢诱发。消融心房左侧或右侧 GP 能显著增加同侧或对侧肺静脉和心房的房颤阈值。自主神经阻滞剂（艾司洛尔或阿托品）显著提高所有部位的房颤阈值。

2. 刺激 SVC-Ao GP 相对选择性的缩短 SVC 的 ERP 和增加 SVC 的 WOV。消融 SVC-Ao GP 仅能延长 SVC 的 ERP、减小 SVC 的 WOV 和消除 SVC 起源的 rapid firing。消融其它 GP 不能抑制 SVC 起源的 rapid firing。

3. 心耳表面应用 Ach 后，心耳出现快速而规则的电激动并驱动房颤。越靠近 GP 的部位，CFAE 越明显。GP 消融后，CFAE 明显减少并且分布梯度消失。在脂肪垫内注入 Ach 后，GP 周围出现显著的 CFAE 并出现同样的梯度，GP 消融过程中，绝大多数房颤中止。

4. 心耳快速起搏引起急性心房电重构，表现为 ERP 缩短和 WOV 不断增宽。GP 消融能逆转和阻止心耳快速起搏诱发的急性心房电重构。

结论：1. 心房和肺静脉的自主神经末梢兴奋通过激活心脏内在自主神经网络，诱发 rapid firing 和 rapid firing 介导的房颤。GP 消融可以抑制 rapid firing 和房颤的发生。

2. SVC-Ao GP 相对选择性调控 SVC 的电生理性质。消融 SVC-Ao GP 可以抑制 SVC 起源的 rapid firing。

3. 心脏内在自主神经系统在 CFAE 的发生机制中发挥了重要作用，GP 消融能减少或消除 CFAE。

4. 心脏内在自主神经系统的激活可能是导致急性心房电重构的重要机制，GP 消融能逆转和阻止快速起搏诱发的急性心房电重构。

关键词：心房颤动；自主神经系统；肺静脉；上腔静脉；碎裂电位；电重构

Abstract

Clinical studies reported that most paroxysmal atrial fibrillation (AF) was due to rapid firing originating from pulmonary veins (PVs) or superior vena cava (SVC). Radiofrequency ablation for isolating PVs or SVC can reduce or prevent AF recurrence. Previous investigations have focused on the mechanism underlying rapid firing originating from PVs or SVC from histological and electrophysiological aspects. However, the results of numerous *in vivo* and *in vitro* studies on this subject have not conclusively defined a mechanism. Several studies suggested that PV isolation is not absolutely necessary for eliminating AF since ablation strategies targeting complex fractionated atrial electrograms (CFAE) or ganglionated plexus (GP) with PV or SVC potentials preserved are also effective. A clear understanding of the respective role of PV, SVC, CFAE and GP in the mechanisms for AF is extremely important for establishing the best target for AF ablation. Our previous studies indicated that the intrinsic cardiac autonomic nervous system is involved in the initiation of AF. Clinical data also reported that GP ablation can prevent paroxysmal AF and even chronic AF with significant atrial electrical remodeling in some patients. In this serial of experiments, the autonomic mechanisms for rapid firing, CFAE and atrial electrical remodeling were studied.

Aims: 1. To investigate the autonomic mechanism for rapid firing originating from PVs and atrial sites.

2. To investigate the autonomic mechanism for rapid firing originating from SVC.

3. To investigate the autonomic mechanism for CFAE.

4. To investigate the autonomic mechanism for acute atrial electrical remodeling induced by rapid pacing.

Methods: Adult healthy mongrel dogs weighing 20 ~ 25 kg were used. The chest was entered via a left or right thoracotomy at the 4th intercostal space. Multi-electrode catheters were sutured to allow recording and stimulation at the left and right PVs, both atria and atrial appendages (AA). A ring (Lasso) catheter was advanced into the SVC for recording and stimulation via the right jugular vein. Left and right vago-sympathetic trunks were isolated for stimulation. All tracings from the electrode catheters were amplified and digitally recorded.

1. High-frequency electrical stimulation (HFS, 200Hz) coupled to each S1S1 (cycle length = 330 msec) pacing stimulus was delivered within myocardial refractoriness to selectively stimulate local neural elements at each site. The lowest HFS voltage at which AF was induced, i. e., AF threshold, was determined before and after (1) ablation of ipsolateral or contralateral GP and (2) administration of autonomic blockers, esmolol or atropine.

2. The effective refractoriness period (ERP) and window of vulnerability (WOV) of AF were determined during stimulation and after ablation of the GP in "the 3rd fat pad" (SVC-Ao GP). Rapid firing was induced by HFS within myocardial refractoriness at the SVC sleeves. The inducibility of rapid firing by HFS was measured after ablation of the SVC-Ao GP or the major atrial GP.

3. Sustained AF was induced by local application of acetylcholine (Ach 10, 100 mM) to the surface of the AA or by injection of Ach (10 mM) into the fat pads containing GP. The extent and degree of CFAE on the atrium were measured before and after ablation of ipsolateral GP.

4. Rapid pacing (1200 bpm) was delivered at the left atrial appendage for 6 hours before and after ablation of the major atrial GP. ERP and WOV were measured at each site during each pacing hour and after

GP ablation.

Results: 1. Rapid firing-mediated AF was induced by local HFS during myocardial refractoriness at each site. Ablation of left or right-sided GP on the atria significantly increased AF threshold at ipsolateral and contralateral PVs, atrium and atrial appendage. Administration of esmolol (1 mg/kg) or atropine (1 mg), significantly elevated AF threshold at all sites.

2. HFS of the SVC-Ao GP induced more significant shortening of ERP and a greater increase in WOV at the SVC than other sites. Ablation of the SVC-Ao GP significantly increased the baseline ERP and decreased the baseline WOV only at the SVC. Rapid firing mediated-AF induced at SVC by HFS was eliminated by ablation of the SVC-Ao GP but was not altered by ablation of the major atrial GP.

3. After AF was induced with Ach either by topical application to the AA or by direct injection into the GP, CFAE exhibited a significant gradient of progressively decreasing dominant frequency (DF) and incidence of CFAE (CFAE%) from the GP toward distant sites while regularity index (RI) progressively decreased in the opposite direction. Ablation of GP markedly attenuated CFAE and eliminated these gradients.

4. In animals with rapid pacing first, ERP was markedly shortened in the first two hours and WOV was progressively widened throughout the 6-hour period. After GP ablation, ERP was significantly longer than before ablation and AF could not be induced at any site. In animals with GP ablation or administration of autonomic blockers first, rapid atrial pacing failed to shorten the ERP, and AF could not be induced in most dogs.

Conclusions: 1. Interconnected atrial autonomic network contributes to the formation of rapid firing from the PV and atrial sites in structurally normal hearts. Autonomic denervation suppresses or eliminates those rapid firings.

2. The SVC-Ao GP not only acts as the "head-stage" for the ex-

trinsic autonomic innervations to the heart, but also preferentially modulates electrophysiological and pathophysiological properties of the SVC sleeves. Ablation of the SVC-Ao GP eliminates rapid firing originating from the SVC.

3. Activation of the intrinsic cardiac autonomic nervous system plays an important role in the genesis of CFAE. Ablation of GP attenuates CFAE and eliminates the CFAE gradients.

4. GP ablation reverses and prevents acute electrical remodeling induced by rapid atrial pacing, suggesting that the intrinsic cardiac autonomic nervous system is crucial for this process. The actions or hyperactivity of the autonomic nervous system itself may be a crucial element in acute atrial remodeling.

Key Words: Atrial fibrillation; autonomic nervous system; pulmonary vein; superior vena cava; complexed fractionated atrial electrograms; electrical remodeling

目　　录

引言 ··· 1

第 1 章　肺静脉和心房起源的快速电激动的自主神经机制 ······ 3
　材料和方法 ··· 4
　　1. 动物模型 ··· 4
　　2. 局部心肌不应期内高频刺激 ································· 4
　　3. GP 消融 ·· 5
　　4. 实验分组和设计 ··· 5
　　5. 组织学染色 ··· 5
　　6. 统计学方法 ··· 6
　结果 ·· 6
　　1. GP 消融前 ·· 6
　　2. GP 消融后 ·· 7
　　3. 组织学染色结果 ··· 7
　讨论 ·· 8
　　1. 主要发现 ·· 8
　　2. Rapid Firing 的发生机制 ····································· 8
　　3. 心脏内在自主神经系统内 GP 的相互作用 ··············· 9
　　4. LOM ·· 10
　　5. 临床意义 ·· 10
　　6. 研究局限性 ··· 10
　结论 ·· 11

第 2 章　上腔静脉起源的快速电激动的自主神经机制 ············ 24
　材料和方法 ··· 24

  1. 动物模型 ······ 24
  2. 程控电刺激 ······ 25
  3. SVC-Ao GP 的刺激和消融方法 ······ 25
  4. 实验设计 ······ 26
  5. HE 染色 ······ 26
  6. 统计学处理 ······ 27
 结果 ······ 27
 讨论 ······ 28
  1. 主要发现 ······ 28
  2. SVC-Ao GP 与上下游结构的联系 ······ 29
  3. SVC Firing 的自主神经机制 ······ 29
  4. 临床意义 ······ 30
  5. 研究局限性 ······ 30
 结论 ······ 30

第3章　心房碎裂电位的自主神经机制 ······ 42
 材料和方法 ······ 42
  1. 动物模型的制备 ······ 42
  2. 实验设计 ······ 43
  3. CFAE 的特点分析 ······ 44
  4. 统计学分析 ······ 45
 结果 ······ 45
  碎裂电位的稳定性 ······ 45
 讨论 ······ 46
  1. 主要发现 ······ 46
  2. 心脏内在自主神经系统和 CFAE 的关系 ······ 47
  3. 心-心反射和房颤 ······ 47
  4. 临床意义 ······ 48
  5. 研究局限性 ······ 48
 结论 ······ 49

第 4 章　房颤致房颤现象的自主神经机制 …… 61
材料和方法 …… 61
　1. 动物模型的制备 …… 61
　2. 快速起搏与程控电刺激 …… 62
　3. GP 消融 …… 62
　4. 自主神经阻滞剂的应用 …… 63
　5. 实验分组和设计 …… 63
　6. 统计学处理 …… 63
结果 …… 64
　1. ERP 和 WOV …… 64
　2. ERP 离散度 …… 64
讨论 …… 65
　1. 主要发现 …… 65
　2. "房颤致房颤"的机制 …… 65
　3. 急性电重构的机制 …… 66
　4. 临床意义 …… 67
　5. 研究的局限性 …… 67
结论 …… 68

第 5 章　综述：心房颤动的发生机制
　　——心脏内在自主神经系统的作用 …… 76
　1. 阵发性房颤的发生机制 …… 76
　2. 慢性房颤的发生机制 …… 78
　3. 心-心反射（Cardio-Cardiac Reflex）与房颤 …… 78
　4. 房颤的射频消融治疗 …… 79
　5. 结论 …… 81

参考文献 …… 82

后记 …… 100

引 言

　　心房颤动(房颤)是临床最常见的快速性心律失常,也是患者致残和致死的重要原因。20世纪末,当临床医生还在争论节律控制、室律控制孰优孰劣的时候,Haissaguerre等[1]发现大多数阵发性房颤起源于肺静脉肌袖内的局灶快速电激动(Rapid Firing);消融这些异位激动灶能减少或阻止房颤的发作。从最初的肺静脉内点状消融到Lasso标测电极指导下的节段性肺静脉隔离,再到Carto导管三维电解剖指导下的环肺静脉消融,技术上的革新带来了成功率的不断提高。然而,在电生理医生普遍关注肺静脉的同时,另有两种代表性的术式——碎裂电位(CFAE)消融[2]和神经节(GP)消融[3]产生,据报道亦能获得类似于甚至高于肺静脉隔离的成功率。尽管目前后两种术式并没有得到电生理界的广泛认同,但是从严格意义上讲对比这几种术式的大规模前瞻性研究并没有出现,因此其优劣并不清楚。对于同一种疾病同时存在着多种不同的治疗手段,本身就说明我们对其发生机制认识上的不足。我们在热衷于比较各种消融术式成功率的同时,不妨冷静的思考:为什么不同的消融靶点(PV、CFAE、GP)同样有效? PV、CFAE、GP三者在房颤的发生机制中扮演什么样的角色?

　　近年来,关于房颤发生机制的研究层出不穷,但是这些研究大多局限于肺静脉特殊的解剖学特点和电生理性质[4~8],得出的结论也仅能解释房颤的某一个方面。以前的研究发现以GP为核心的心脏内在自主神经系统在房颤的发生中占有重要地位[9~12]。本研究以目前房颤导管消融策略中的疑点和难点为线索,通过大体动物模型和电生理标测方法,探讨Rapid Firing、CFAE和心房电重构与心脏内在自主神经系统的关系,试图阐明房颤发生的关键机制,为制定最佳消融策略提供理论依据。具体研究内容如下：
①肺静脉和心房起源的 Rapid Firing 的自主神经机制；
②上腔静脉起源的 Rapid Firing 的自主神经机制；
③CFAE 的自主神经机制；
④心房电重构的自主神经机制。

第1章 肺静脉和心房起源的快速电激动的自主神经机制

近年来，心房颤动（房颤）研究领域的一个重要发现是：大多数阵发性房颤由肺静脉内局灶快速电激动（Rapid Firing）引起[1~3]。尽管有大量研究试图从组织学和电生理学方面寻找Rapid Firing的根源，但是并未获得一致的结论[4~7]。以往的离体动物心脏实验观察到[8~12]，肺静脉Rapid Firing能被自主神经刺激所诱发，被自主神经阻滞剂所抑制，提示肺静脉Rapid Firing可能与心脏自主神经系统有关。

支配心脏的自主神经系统分为外在自主神经系统和内在自主神经系统[13,14]。前者指心包以外的自主神经成分，例如位于颈部的迷走交感干、星状神经节等，后者指心包以内的自主神经成分，主要包括心外膜脂肪垫内的自主神经节（ganglionated plexus，GP）及其发出的神经纤维。解剖学资料表明，心房表面主要的GP包括：①右前GP（ARGP），位于右上肺静脉（RSPV）和右心房（RA）的交界处；②右下GP（IRGP），位于右下肺静脉（RIPV）和下腔静脉的交界处；③左上GP（SLGP），位于左上肺静脉（LSPV）和左肺动脉的交界处；④左下GP（ILGP），位于左下肺静脉（LIPV）和左心房（LA）的交界处。此外，最新的研究发现[15~18]，Marshall韧带（LOM）也含有较多的GP。心房表面的GP不仅仅是外在自主神经系统通向心脏的中继站，而且是窦房结、房室结功能和心房电生理性质的调控中心，有学者称为"微脑"系统[19,20]。

离体组织电生理实验观察到[21]，肺静脉肌袖和心房肌有效不应期内的高频电刺激可以通过兴奋自主神经末梢诱发Rapid Firing，其特点与阵发性房颤患者肺静脉或心房起源的Rapid Firing相似。

本研究中，我们通过消融犬心外膜不同的 GP，系统评价心脏内在自主神经系统在肺静脉或心房起源的 Rapid Firing 的发生机制中的作用。

材料和方法

1．动物模型

正常成年杂种犬共 36 只，体重 20～25kg，以戊巴比妥钠 50mg/kg 麻醉后，气管插管机械通气。分离双侧股动、静脉，分别置入鞘管。右侧股静脉鞘管内送入体温调节仪，使体温维持在 36.5±1.5℃。左侧股静脉用于滴注生理盐水，维持液体平衡。右侧股动脉用于监测动脉血压。左侧股动脉内送入四极标测导管至主动脉根部无冠窦内记录 His 电位。分离双侧颈部迷走交感干。持续记录肢体导联 ECG。

经左侧第四肋间开胸，剪开心包，暴露心脏。将八极电生理记录导管（Biosense-Webster，USA）分别缝于左心耳（LAA）、LA、LSPV 和 LIPV 表面（图 1-1）。同样，经右侧第四肋间开胸，将导管缝于右心耳（RAA）、RA、RSPV 和 RIPV 表面（图 1-1）。所有电生理信号由巴德电生理记录系统（美国巴德公司生产）记录和分析，滤波设置在 30～250Hz。

2．局部心肌不应期内高频刺激

高频电刺激（high frequency stimulation，HFS，图 1-2）在每个心房起搏信号（电压为 2 倍起搏阈值，起搏周长为 330ms）后 2msec 发放。HFS 由一串长度 40ms，频率 200Hz，脉宽 0.1ms，电压 0.6～12V 的脉冲组成（S-88 型双通道刺激仪，美国 Astro-Med 公司生产），保证 HFS 发放在心肌有效不应期内，仅刺激神经成分（图 1-2，图 1-3）[18,21]。一旦 Rapid Firing 产生，HFS 立即停止以便观察能否诱发房颤。根据以前的研究[22]，房颤定义为持续 5s 以上的快速而不规则的心房激动（>500bpm）伴不规则的房室传导（图 1-4）。

房颤的持续时间从 HFS 停止开始计算。房颤阈值为 HFS 能诱发房颤的最低电压。

3. GP 消融

心房 GP 位于心外膜脂肪垫内(图 1-5)。在解剖学定位的基础上,采用快速电刺激(20Hz,0.1ms,1~12V)对 GP 进行精确定位。刺激和消融均采用美国 AtriCure 生产的刺激/消融两用笔进行。快速电刺激时出现心率明显减慢且减慢程度与刺激电压成正比为阳性反应。一旦发现阳性反应,立即由刺激模式转换到消融模式,直接放电消融(图 1-6)。刺激和消融 ARGP、IRGP、SLGP、ILGP 以及 Marshall 韧带内的 GP 均采用以上方法进行。GP 消融部位远离导管记录和刺激部位(图 1-1,图 1-6)。GP 消融有效的标志是在最强电压(12V)刺激情况下所有阳性反应消失,刺激同侧迷走神经也无明显反应。

4. 实验分组和设计

第 1 组:消融 ARGP 和 IRGP 对同侧和对侧肺静脉、心房和心耳部位房颤阈值的影响。同侧包括 RSPV、RIPV、RA 和 RAA,对侧包括 LSPV、LIPV、LA 和 LAA。

第 2 组:消融 SLGP、ILGP 和 LOM 对同侧和对侧肺静脉、心房和心耳部位房颤阈值的影响。同侧包括 LSPV、LIPV、LA 和 LAA,对侧包括 RSPV、RIPV、RA 和 RAA。

第 3 组:静脉推注自主神经阻滞剂、艾司洛尔(esmolol,1mg/kg)或阿托品(atropine,1mg),对肺静脉、心房和心耳部位房颤阈值的影响。

5. 组织学染色

HE 染色:对 5 条犬(4 条消融犬和 1 条对照犬)的 ARGP 进行了 HE 染色。包含 ARGP 的脂肪垫和临近的心房肌被切下并固定在中性福尔马林溶液中 24h。石蜡包埋后,在组织横截面切片,按照常规 HE 染色方法染色。

免疫组织化学染色：对未消融的对照犬进行免疫组织化学染色观察自主神经成分。分别采用胆碱能神经系统特异性抗体-酪氨酸羟化酶(tyrosine hydroxylase，TH)抗体和肾上腺素能神经系统特异性抗体-胆碱乙酰转移酶(choline acetyl transferase，ChAT)抗体，按照常规方法对组织进行染色。

6. 统计学方法

由于存在房颤无法诱发的情况，本研究中房颤阈值采用四分位数表示(表1-1 ~ 表1-4)。GP消融或应用自主神经阻滞剂前后房颤阈值的变化采用非参数 Wilcoxon 符号等级检验法进行比较。$P < 0.05$ 为有统计学差异。

结　果

1. GP消融前

心房 S1S1 起搏的阈值平均为 0.2 ± 0.05 V(消融后未改变)。心肌不应期内的 HFS 可使起搏条件下的 AH 间期延长和使房颤过程中 AV 传导减慢，在肺静脉多见。如图 1-2A 所示，当在 LSPV 发放 1.5V 的 HFS 时，可见 AH 间期明显延长并出现 2:1 AV 传导阻滞。在图 2B 中，在 LIPV 发放 2.4V 的 HFS 诱发房颤，在房颤发生前出现 AV 阻滞，房颤过程中可见 AV 传导减慢或阻滞。以上现象说明了自主神经被心肌不应期内的 HFS 充分激活。

GP 消融前，Rapid Firing 介导的房颤能被发放在各个部位的 HFS(心肌不应期内)反复诱发。HFS 停止后，随着自主神经张力的逐渐下降，房颤随之中止。如图 1-3B、图 1-4 和图 1-7 所示，Firing 大多起源于刺激位点，前 10 个激动波的平均周期为 55 ± 15 ms。房颤的平均持续时间为 8 ± 5 s。

所有 Firing 的第一个激动波发生于高频刺激停止后的 30 ~ 160 ms(图 1-3、图 1-4、图 1-7)，即发生在相邻两串 HFS 中间，而并非紧跟 HFS 的最后一个脉冲信号，这说明 Rapid Firing 并非由直接的心肌刺激(即 HFS 脱离心肌不应期)所引起。为了进一步验证，我们将 HFS 的持续时间由 40ms 缩短到 20ms，结果仍然能诱发房颤，但是刺激电压稍高。以上现象表明，本实验中采用的 HFS 达到了心肌不应期内有效刺激自主神经的目的。

2. GP 消融后

第 1 组(表 1-1)：消融 ARGP 和 IRGP 后，房颤阈值在 RA、RAA、RSPV 和 RIPV 部位显著增高。消融这两个 GP 后，9 条犬 (9/14) 的 RSPV 以及 10 条犬的 RIPV (10/14) 即使用最高电压 (12V) 亦不能诱发 Rapid Firing 和房颤。房颤仍然能在 RA(13/14) 和 RAA(10/10) 部位被 HFS 诱发但阈值升高。消融 ARGP 和 IRGP 后，对侧部位(LAA、LA、LSPV 和 LIPV)的房颤阈值也显著升高。

第 2 组(表 1-2 和表 1-3)：消融 SLGP 和 ILGP 以后，同侧 (LAA、LA、LSPV 和 LIPV)和对侧(RAA、RA 和 RSPV)部位的房颤阈值均显著增高(表 1-2)。继续消融位于 LOM 的 GP 后，左侧部位的房颤阈值进一步升高(表 1-3)。

我们对其中的 6 只犬消融心房上所有的 GP(ARGP + IRGP + SLGP + ILGP + LOM)后，即使采用最大电压，HFS 依然不能在任何肺静脉诱发 Rapid Firing 和房颤(图 1-7)，但是仍然能在心房(4/6)或心耳部位(4/6)诱发，但是阈值显著升高(P 均小于 0.05)。

第 3 组(表 1-4)：静脉推注 esmolol (1mg/kg)后房颤阈值在所有测量部位均显著增加；静脉推注 atropine (1 mg)后，房颤在任何部位均不能被诱发。

3. 组织学染色结果

HE 染色：如图 1-8 所示，脂肪垫内含有大量神经节细胞。GP 消融后，这些神经节被严重破坏，周边心房肌基本没有受到损伤。

免疫组织化学染色：如图 1-9 所示，GP 内既含有大量副交感神经元(ChaT 阳性，图 1-8A 和图 1-8B)，也含有一定量的交感神经成分(TH 阳性，图 1-9C 和图 1-9D)。

讨 论

1. 主要发现

本研究观察到，Rapid Firing 介导的房颤能通过高频刺激自主神经末梢诱发。消融心房左侧或右侧 GP 显著增加同侧或对侧肺静脉和心房结构的房颤阈值（表 1-1 和表 1-2）。消融 LOM 内的 GP 进一步提高左侧肺静脉和心房结构的房颤阈值（表 1-3）。自主神经阻滞剂（esmolol 或 atropine）能显著增加所有部位的房颤阈值（表 1-4）。以上现象证实了紧密相连的心脏内在自主神经网络参与了肺静脉和心房起源的 Focal Firing 的发生机制。

2. Rapid Firing 的发生机制

肺静脉 Rapid Firing 的发生机制目前尚不清楚。自律性增加、触发活动和微折返分别被部分学者认为与 Rapid Firing 的产生有关。尽管有组织学证据表明[5]，肺静脉内存在着起搏样细胞——P 细胞，其异常增加的自律性可能是 Firing 产生的机制，但以下现象不支持这一假设：①这些 P 细胞存在于肺静脉的远端，而 Firing 产生于肺静脉的近端；②舒张期除极是自律性电活动的特征性现象，然而有研究观察到 Firing 起始前并不存在舒张期除极[12]；③离体灌流的肺静脉肌袖并未观察到自发的电活动[23]，即使存在也非常微弱；④迷走神经兴奋抑制自律性却有助于房颤的发生；⑤肺静脉电隔离术时，阻断肺静脉和心房之间的电连接从理论上不会影响肺静脉内的自律性，然而在绝大多数情况下 Firing 中止。动物房颤模型的光学标测结果提示微折返可能是 Firing 的维持机制[24]，但微折返大多是在灌注迷走神经递质乙酰胆碱（Ach）或有明显心房组织结构改变的基础上由一个或多个快速电活动所诱发，微折返从来不会自发产生。临床研究中，应用高密度电极标测阵发性房颤患者的肺静脉发现[25]：微折返虽然存在但并不持续，不是维持 Firing 和房颤所必需。

Patterson 等[8,9]在研究离体灌流的犬肺静脉-心房组织电生理特点时发现,触发活动可能是产生 Firing 的机制。Firing 可被海豚毒素、阿托品或者阿替洛尔抑制,表明迷走成分和交感成分均参与了 Firing 的形成。作者推测心脏内在自主神经兴奋导致神经末梢释放胆碱能递质(Ach)和肾上腺素能递质(NE)。前者导致心肌不应期缩短,后者通过提升细胞内的钙离子浓度增加早后除极,Firing 在二者的共同作用下形成。为了验证这一推测,Patterson 等在肺静脉肌袖的灌流液中加入低浓度的 Ach 和 NE,结果诱发了高频快速电活动,类似于临床观察到的 Rapid Firing。随后的光学标测结果进一步支持触发活动是诱发 Firing 的机制[12]。本研究中,我们通过选择性刺激自主神经末梢诱发了 Firing,可能的机制是:局部自主神经末梢受到刺激后不仅能在局部直接释放贮存的神经递质,而且能通过传入纤维激活 GP 并进一步释放递质。由于 GP 内既含有大量的副交感神经元又含有部分交感神经成分(图 1-9)[26],因此释放的递质里既含 Ach 又含 NE,二者为 Firing 的产生提供了条件。GP 消融或自主神经阻滞后,Firing 难以诱发,进一步证实了自主神经系统在 Firing 产生中的重要作用。

3. 心脏内在自主神经系统内 GP 的相互作用

以前的研究发现,心脏内在自主神经系统内的 GP 通过神经连接形成了一个紧密相连的网络,调节窦房结和房室结功能。本研究支持以上发现。如图 1-3 所示,选择性刺激位于 LSPV 和 LIPV 的自主神经末梢能显著抑制右侧的房室结传导功能,表明局部神经末梢的兴奋能通过神经传导激活整个心脏自主神经系统。本研究中,消融心房左侧或右侧 GP,不仅使临近的肺静脉和心房的房颤诱发性降低,而且能提高对侧肺静脉和心房结构的房颤阈值,证实了紧密相连的内在自主神经网络在房颤诱发中的重要作用。以前的研究也有类似发现:刺激房颤患者的 GP 能在 4~5cm 以外的对侧肺静脉产生快速紊乱的电活动[27]。在犬右侧的 ARGP 内注入微量的 Ach 能在对侧的 LSPV 产生 Rapid Firing[10]。本试验中,如图 1-4 所示,发放在 LAA 的 HFS 诱发了 Rapid Firing,但仅持续 1~2s 后,起源于左侧肺静脉的 Firing 接替 LAA 成为房颤驱动灶。这种现象进一步提示整个心脏内在自主神经网络被局部的高频刺激充分激活。肺静脉与 GP 的毗邻关系及肺静脉对自主神经递质的敏感性使其成为驱动房颤的活跃成分。

4. LOM

组织学和电生理学研究显示，交感和迷走成分均存在于 LOM。本研究观察到，消融 LOM 内的 GP 能进一步增加左侧肺静脉和左心房的房颤阈值(表1-3)。这一现象与 Doshi 等[17]和 Lin 等[18]的研究结果一致，说明了 LOM 是心脏内在自主神经网络的重要组成部分，并且在 Firing 的发生机制中发挥了重要作用。

5. 临床意义

临床研究发现，大部分心脏结构正常的阵发性房颤由肺静脉起源的 Rapid Firing 所驱动，其具体机制不清。本研究中，Rapid Firing 介导的房颤能被较低电压的局部自主神经刺激轻易诱发，并且能被 GP 消融所抑制，提示了心脏内在自主神经网络的激活可能是阵发性房颤患者肺静脉 Rapid Firing 产生的重要机制。本实验的对象是在正常成年犬，因此本实验结果可能适用于临床观察到的心脏结构正常的阵发性房颤。临床消融资料表明，肺静脉隔离术对大部分阵发性房颤患者有效[2,3]。Lemery 等[28]的研究发现，即使放电消融时未出现明显的迷走反射，环肺静脉消融仍然能使 88% 迷走反射阳性位点去神经支配，提示环肺静脉消融径线已经包含了大部分 GP 所在区域，环肺静脉消融所获得的成功率可能跟不自觉地消融 GP 有一定关系。此外，至少对于有明确自主神经机制参与的阵发性房颤患者，损伤范围更小、靶点更明确的 GP 消融可能是一个更好的选择。

6. 研究局限性

本研究中，选择性刺激心房和肺静脉局部的自主神经成分诱发 Rapid Firing，我们推测副交感和交感系统都参与这一过程，但是没有直接证据证明交感系统被激活。然而，β受体阻滞剂艾司洛尔能使所有部位的房颤阈值显著提高，间接提示交感系统的重要性。由于副交感系统对外界刺激因素反应迅速而交感神经系统反应缓慢，这是本研究中高频刺激首先观察到副交感激活的原因(图1-3)。

结　　论

本研究通过选择性刺激心房和肺静脉局部的自主神经成分激活了心脏内在自主神经网络，诱发了Rapid Firing和Rapid Firing介导的房颤。GP消融可以抑制这些Rapid Firing的发生。这些研究结果提示了心脏内在自主神经网络在阵发性房颤的发生机制中发挥了重要作用。

表 1-1　消融 ARGP 和 IRGP 对同侧和对侧心房和肺静脉房颤阈值的影响

	同侧					对侧			
	RAA N=14	RA N=10	RSPV N=14	RIPV N=14	LAA N=7	LA N=7	LSPV N=7	LIPV N=7
ARGP+IRGP 消融前	1.5 (1.5; 2.4)	1.5 (1.5; 4.5)	2.4 (2.2; 6.5)	3.2 (2.2; 7.5)	1.5 (1.5; 2.4)	1.5 (1.5; 3.2)	3.2 (3.2; 7)	2.4 (1.5; 6)
ARGP+IRGP 消融后	2.4 (2.2; 5.8)	2.8 (2.2; 6.5)	>12* (9.6; >12)	>12 (11.3; >12)	3.2 (1.5; >12)	4.5 (1.5; >12)	9.5 (4.5; >12)	11.2 (3.2; >12)
P值	<0.01	<0.05	<0.01	<0.01	<0.05	<0.05	<0.05	<0.05

房颤阈值采用四分位数表示,括号内为第 1 四分位和第 3 四分位。GP 消融前后房颤阈值的变化采用非参数 Wilcoxon 符号等级检验法进行比较。*：>12,指即使使用最高电压(12V)也不能诱发房颤。

表 1-2　消融 SLGP 和 ILGP 对同侧和对侧心房和肺静脉房颤阈值的影响

	同 侧				对 侧			
	LAA N=10	LA N=6	LSPV N=10	LIPV N=10	RAA N=10	RA N=8	RSPV N=10	RIPV N=10
SLGP+ILGP 消融前	1.5 (1.5;3.3)	2.8 (2.2;4.5)	2.4 (2.2;2.6)	2.8 (2.2;4.8)	1.5 (1.5;1.8)	1.5 (1.4;1.5)	2.8 (1.5;9)	3.8 (2.2;9)
SLGP+ILGP 消融后	3.8 (2.2;8)	8.5 (4.5;9.5)	8 (3.2;11.2)	9.5 (3.2;>12)	2.8 (1.9;3.2)	2.4 (1.8;4.8)	6.5 (4.5;9.8)	7 (4.5;9.2)
P 值	<0.01	<0.05	<0.01	<0.01	<0.05	<0.05	<0.01	0.2

表 1-3　消融 Marshall 韧带（LOM）对左侧心房和肺静脉房颤阈值的影响

	LAA (N=9)	LA (N=6)	LSPV (N=9)	LIPV (N=9)
SLGP+ILGP 消融后	3.2 (2; 9.3)	8.5 (4.5; 9.5)	8 (3.2; 9.6)	9.6 (5.2; >12)
SLGP+ILGP+LOM 消融后	8 (4; 11.6)	>12 (6.7; >12)	>12 (8; >12)	>12 (11; >12)
P 值	<0.05	<0.05	<0.05	<0.05

第1章 肺静脉和心房起源的快速电激动的自主神经机制

表1-4　应用自主神经阻滞剂后对心房和肺静脉房颤阈值的影响

		LAA	LA	LSPV	LIPV	RAA	RA	RSPV	RIPV
Atropine ($N=5$)									
	Before	2.4 (1.5; 2.4)	1.5 (1.5; 4)	3.2 (1.5; 3.2)	2.4 (1.5; 2.4)	1.5 (1.5; 2.4)	1.5 (1.5; 2.6)	2.4 (2; 6.5)	4.5 (2.4; 9.3)
	After	>12	>12	>12	>12	>12	>12	>12	>12
	P value	<0.05	<0.05	<0.05	<0.05	<0.05	<0.05	<0.05	<0.05
Esmolol ($N=7$)									
	Before	1.5 (1.5; 2.4)	1.5 (1.4; 2.4)	3.2 (1.5; 6)	3.2 (2.4; 4.5)	1.5 (1.5; 2.4)	2.4 (1.5; 4.5)	3.2 (2.4; 3.2)	3.2 (2.4; 8)
	After	4.5 (3.2; 6)	4.5 (3.2; 6)	6 (4.5; 9)	8 (7; 10.4)	4.5 (2.4; 6)	6 (3.2; 7)	6 (3.2; 6)	6 (4.5; 9)
	P value	<0.05	<0.05	<0.05	<0.05	<0.05	<0.05	<0.05	<0.05

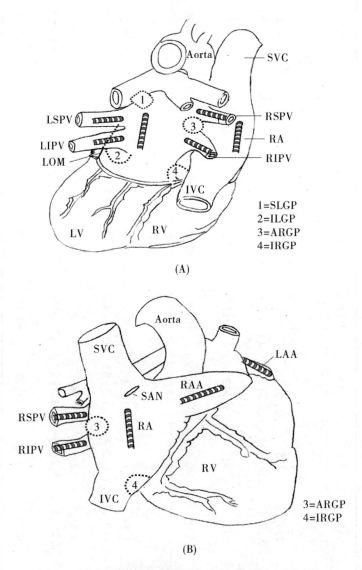

图1-1 电生理导管的记录部位以及心房主要 GP 所在位置。(A) 后前位;(B) 右侧位。SLGP:左上 GP;ILGP:左下 GP;ARGP:右前 GP;IRGP:右下 GP;SVC:上腔静脉;IVC:下腔静脉;SAN:窦房结;LOM:Marshall 韧带。

第1章 肺静脉和心房起源的快速电激动的自主神经机制

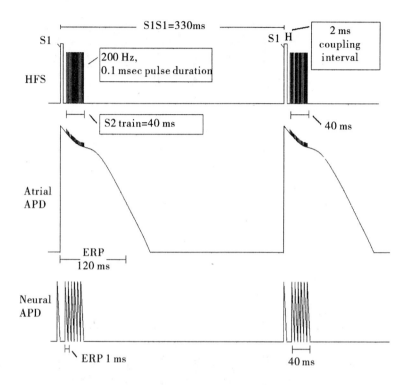

图1-2 心肌不应期内高频刺激(HFS)示意图。

心房肌在2倍起搏阈电压下的有效不应期(ERP)大约为120ms,而神经ERP仅为1ms左右,考虑到在自主神经刺激条件下心房肌ERP会缩短,因此将HFS的时限设为40me,以确保刺激在心肌不应期内。HFS在基础起搏的每个S1刺激信号后2ms发放,刺激频率为200Hz,脉宽为0.1ms,电压为0.6~12V。

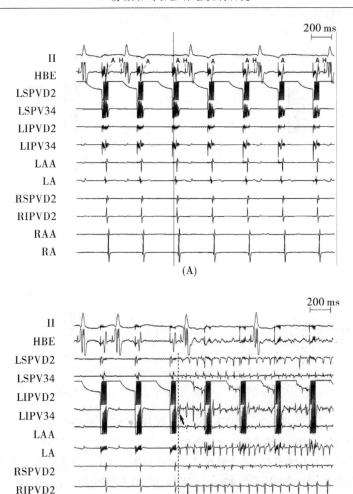

图1-3 心肌不应期内高频刺激(HFS)抑制AV传导。
(A)在LSPV发放1.5V的HFS时出现AH间期延长和2∶1 AV传导阻滞;
(B)在LIPV发放2.4V的HFS诱发房颤,起源于刺激部位(箭头)。房颤发生前出现AV传导阻滞,房颤过程中高频刺激明显抑制AV传导。这些现象说明自主神经被HFS充分激活。

第1章 肺静脉和心房起源的快速电激动的自主神经机制

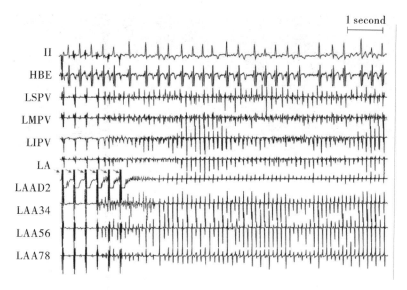

图1-4　在左心耳(LAA)心肌不应期内发放高频刺激(箭头)
诱发Rapid Firing和Rapid Firing介导的房颤

在本图中,起源于LAA的Rapid Firing诱发了房颤,但起源于左侧肺静脉尤其是LMPV的Rapid Firing很快接替LAA驱动房颤,间接提示了整个自主神经系统被激活,具体见讨论部分。

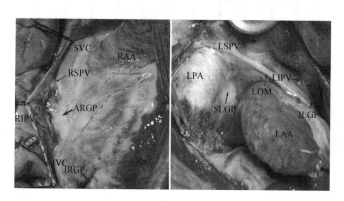

图1-5　心房主要GP所在部位
ARGP：右前GP；IRGP：右下GP；SLGP：左上GP；ILGP：左下GP。其它简称同图1-1。

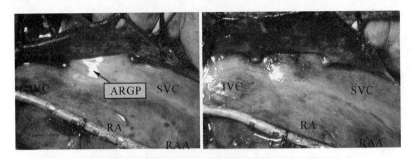

图1-6 ARGP消融前后

GP消融采用刺激/消融两用笔,刺激时一旦发现窦率减缓或房室传导阻滞,立即由刺激模式转换为消融模式放电消融,直至周边所有部位对刺激的反应消失。右图中消融区域局限,对周边心肌组织影响较小。

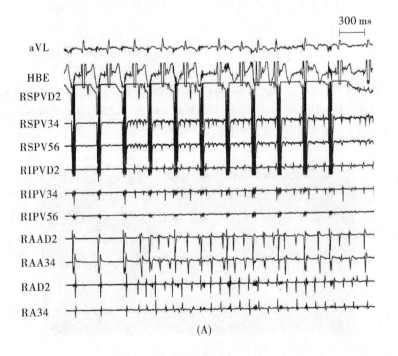

(A)

第1章　肺静脉和心房起源的快速电激动的自主神经机制

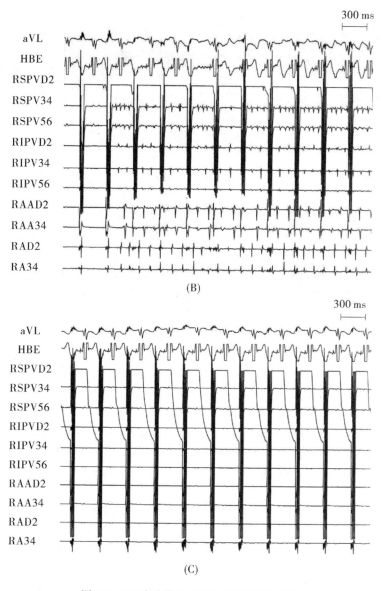

图1-7　GP消融前后RSPV房颤阈值的变化

(A)GP消融前，在RSPV心肌不应期内发放1.5V的高频刺激诱发Rapid Firing和Rapid Firing介导的房颤；(B)消融RSPV同侧GP，即ARGP和IRGP后，房颤阈值增高为9.3V；(C)继续消融对侧GP，即SLGP、ILGP和LOM后，最大电压(12V)的高频刺激在RSPV也不能Rapid Firing和房颤。

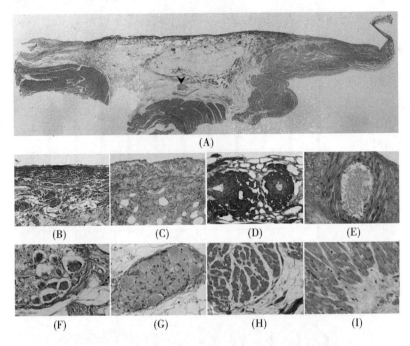

图 1-8 消融犬和正常对照犬 ARGP 的 HE 染色结果

放大倍数分别为(A)1X,(B)和(C)20X,(D)至(I)40X。图(A)、(B)、(D)、(F)和(H)取自 GP 消融犬,图(C)、(E)、(G)、(I)取自正常对照犬。(A)消融范围。紫色中央区域为消融后坏死灶,周边区域为未受损的心肌组织。箭头指向消融后的神经节;(B)GP 消融后,心外膜下胶原纤维变成深紫色,失去组织学形态;(C)正常对照犬的胶原纤维作为对照;(D)GP 消融后,小血管壁变成深紫色,失去组织学形态;(E)正常对照犬的小血管作为对照;(F)图 A 中箭头所指的神经节,神经元胞体结构皱缩,周围残留大量空泡,这些都是坏死的组织学特征;(G)正常对照犬的 GP 作为对照;(H)GP 消融后,尽管周边胶原纤维受损,但是临近心肌并没有发生明显变化;(I)正常对照犬的心肌作为对照。

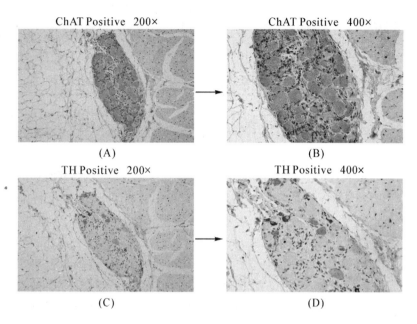

图1-9 免疫组织化学染色

棕色区域为阳性区域。各图中左侧为脂肪组织,中间椭圆形为 GP,右侧为心肌组织。(A,B) ChAT 阳性,胆碱能神经系统特异性标志,可见 ChAT 阳性神经元几乎布满整个 GP;(C,D) TH 阳性,肾上腺素能神经系统特异性标志,可见 TH 阳性神经元散在分布。

第 2 章 上腔静脉起源的快速电激动的自主神经机制

临床上,部分阵发性房颤患者的 Rapid Firing 位于肺静脉以外,以上腔静脉(SVC)最为常见[1]。有研究发现,起源于 SVC 的 Rapid Firing 多位于后壁[2],与上腔静脉-主动脉 GP(SVC-Ao GP)相邻。SVC-Ao GP 位于 SVC、右肺动脉(RPA)和主动脉(Ao)交界处的脂肪垫内。应用高频电流刺激此部位,可以明显减慢心率和抑制房室传导[3~5]。含有 SVC-Ao GP 的脂肪垫又称为"第三脂肪垫",被认为是外在迷走神经通向心脏的中继站[5]。以前的研究提示了自主神经机制参与了 Rapid Firing 的形成[6~10]。在本书第 1 章我们发现,消融心房表面的 GP 可以抑制起源于肺静脉和心房部位的 Rapid Firing。由于 SVC 和 SVC-Ao GP 的毗邻关系,我们推测 SVC 起源的 Rapid Firing 可能跟 SVC-Ao GP 有关。本研究中,我们探讨①SVC-Ao GP 与外在自主神经系统以及下游心房结构电生理性质之间的联系;②SVC 起源的 Rapid Firing 的发生机制以及消融 SVC-Ao GP 的影响。

材料和方法

1. 动物模型

正常成年杂种犬共 30 只,体重 20~25kg,以戊巴比妥钠 50mg/kg 麻醉后,气管插管机械通气。分离双侧股动、静脉,分别置入鞘管。右侧股静脉鞘管内送入体温调节仪,使体温维持在 36.5±1.5℃。左侧股静脉用于滴注生理盐水,维持液体平衡。右侧股动脉用于监测动脉血压。左侧股动脉内送入四极标测导管至主动脉根部无冠窦记录 His 电位。持续记录肢体导联 ECG。

经左侧第四肋间开胸，剪开心包，暴露心脏。将多极电生理记录导管缝于 LAA、LA、LSPV 和 LIPV 表面(图2-1)。经右侧第四肋间开胸，将导管缝于 RAA、RA、RSPV 和 RIPV 表面(图 2-1)。分离颈静脉，插入 10F 鞘管，经鞘管送入环状电极导管(Lasso)至 SVC 和 RA 交界以上并固定，记录 SVC 肌袖的电活动。分离双侧颈部迷走交感干，分别插入用绝缘材料包裹的直径 0.1mm 的银丝电极以便于刺激。

2. 程控电刺激

程控电刺激由程控刺激仪发放(Medtronic Inc, USA)。各记录部位的 ERP 采用 S1S2 递减的方法测量：S1－S1＝330ms，S1:S2＝8:1，刺激电压分别采用 2 倍起搏阈值(2×TH)和 10 倍起搏阈值(10×TH)。S1S2 从 150ms 递减，步长 10ms，当遇到不应期时，从上一个 S1S2 间期起，步长减为 1ms 以便精确测量。诱发房颤的难易程度采用心房易颤窗口(window of vulnerability, WOV)的大小来衡量[11]。在 ERP 测量过程中，如果 S1S2 刺激诱发了房颤，那么紧接着测量能诱发房颤的最长和最短 S1S2 间期，二者之差为 WOV。WOV 的值越大表示房颤越容易被诱发，WOV＝0 表示房颤不能被诱发。依据以往研究[11]，房颤定义为持续 5s 以上的快速不规则的心房激动(＞500bpm)伴不规则房室传导。对于 SVC，在 Lasso 电极中选择记录电位较好的多对(平均 3±1 对)电极进行测量，取平均值作为 SVC 的 ERP 和 WOV。

3. SVC-Ao GP 的刺激和消融方法

SVC-Ao GP 的准确部位采用肺动脉逆行途径确定(图2-1)。具体方法是：右侧开胸后，分离与 RSPV 并行的右肺动脉分支，远端结扎，近端穿刺并插入短鞘管。在 X 线透视指导下，通过短鞘管送入篮状电极导管(Biosense-Webster, Diamond Bar, CA)至右肺动脉、SVC 和主动脉交界区附近。篮状电极由首尾相连的 5 根轴组成，每根轴上含等间距的6个电极，每两个相邻的电极可以组成电极对发放电刺激。高频电刺激（频率20Hz，脉宽0.1ms，电压0.6～12V）依次从篮状电极的每个电极对（共25对）发放，引起窦性心率和房室传导最大程度下降的部位为SVC-Ao GP的中心部位。

SVC-Ao GP同样可以通过直视在RPA、SVC和Ao的交界区寻找（图2-2），并通过刺激/消融笔（AtriCure，West Chester，OH）发放高频电刺激确认。刺激SVC-Ao GP可以导致窦性心率和/或房室传导明显减慢。一旦发现阳性反应，立即由刺激模式转换为消融模式。射频能量通过刺激/消融笔在周边所有阳性部位发放，直至最大电压（12V）亦不能减慢窦性心率或房室传导。

4. 实验设计

实验1：分别在基础状态下、同侧颈部迷走交感干刺激和SVC-Ao GP刺激（篮状电极）条件下，测量LA、LAA、LSPV、LIPV、RA、RAA、RSPV、RIPV和SVC部位$2\times TH$和$10\times TH$条件下的ERP和WOV。"同侧"指测量部位的同侧，比如测量LSPV的ERP和WOV时刺激左侧迷走交感干，而测量SVC的ERP和WOV时刺激右侧迷走交感干。同侧迷走交感干刺激和SVC-Ao GP刺激的电压分别设定在导致窦性心率下降50%或能引起2：1房室传导阻滞所需电压。消融SVC-Ao GP后，重复测量以上各部位的ERP和WOV，同侧迷走神经刺激和SVC-Ao GP刺激的电压与消融前相同。

实验2：在SVC肌袖不应期内发放高频刺激[12,13]。具体方法为：在SVC进行恒定的S1S1起搏（2倍起搏阈电压，起搏周长为330ms）。在每个S1起搏信号后2ms发放高频刺激（HFS）。HFS由一串频率200Hz，脉宽0.1ms，时限40ms，电压0.6～12V的脉冲组成（S-88型双通道刺激仪，美国Astro-Med公司生产），确保在心肌不应期内选择性刺激神经成分[12,13]。示意图见论文第1章的图1-2。测量HFS诱发房颤所需的最低电压，即房颤阈值。观察消融SVC-Ao GP或心房表面主要GP后房颤阈值的变化。

5. HE染色

对另外4只未经过消融的正常犬进行组织学染色。在篮状电极和刺激/消融笔发放高频刺激产生最大效果的部位，即 SVC-Ao GP 所在部位取下组织，浸泡于中性福尔马林溶液中 24h。石蜡包埋后，在组织横截面和纵切面切片，按照常规 HE 染色方法染色并观察。

6. 统计学处理

实验 1：配对 T 检验用来比较 SVC-Ao GP 消融前后 ERP 和 WOV 的变化。重复测量的方差分析用来分别比较消融前和消融后基础状态下、SVC-Ao GP 刺激和迷走交感干刺激三者之间 ERP 和 WOV 的差异。

实验 2：非参数统计方法 Wilcoxon 符号等级检验用来比较不同 GP 消融后房颤阈值的变化。

$P < 0.05$ 为差异有显著性。

结　　果

通过篮状电极发放高频刺激的方法，SVC-Ao GP 在 30 只犬均顺利定位。图 2-2 显示其大体解剖形态及周边结构。图 2-3 的 HE 染色结果显示其微观形态：从横切面或纵切面可见众多的神经节细胞聚集于 RPA 附近的浅表脂肪组织下。刺激 SVC-Ao GP 使窦性心率降低 50% 或出现 2:1 房室传导阻滞所需要的电压平均为 $3.5 \pm 0.8V$。刺激左侧或右侧颈部迷走交感干使窦性心率降低 50% 或出现 2:1 房室传导所需要的电压分别为 $1.5 \pm 0.5V$ 和 $1.8 \pm 0.7V$。

实验 1：SVC-Ao GP 消融前（图 2-4），刺激同侧颈部迷走交感干使所有测量部位的 ERP（$2 \times$ 和 $10 \times TH$）明显缩短。刺激 SVC-Ao GP 同样能显著缩短部分位点的 ERP（$2 \times TH$：LSPV、RA、RSPV 和 SVC；$10 \times TH$：LAA、RA 和 SVC），在 SVC 最为显著。一个有趣而重要的发现是：在 SVC，刺激 SVC-Ao GP 引起 ERP 缩短的程度较刺激右侧迷走交感干更为显著（图 2-4 中 $2 \times$ 和 $10 \times TH$ 的 ERP，红色星号标记）；而其它位点情况却恰好相反。WOV 的变化进一步显示 SVC-Ao GP 刺激对 SVC 的相对选择性：刺激同侧颈部迷走交感干能使所有部位的 WOV 增宽，但刺激 SVC-Ao GP 仅能使 SVC 的 WOV 显著增宽。

SVC-Ao GP 消融后（图 2-5），各部位的起搏阈值没有发生明显变化，但是基础状态下的 ERP（2×和 10×TH）仅在 SVC 明显增加，基础状态下的 WOV（10×TH）也仅在 SVC 明显减小，基础状态下的 ERP 和 WOV 在其它部位均无明显变化（表 2-1）。SVC-Ao GP 消融后，以与消融前相同的电压分别刺激左右侧颈部迷走交感干不能减慢心率和 AV 传导，也不能使 ERP 和 WOV 发生明显改变，但是以最大电压刺激左右侧颈部迷走交感干仍然能使心率和 AV 传导轻度减慢。

实验 2：为了进一步验证 SVC-Ao GP 与起源于 SVC 的 Rapid Firing 的关系，我们在 SVC 肌袖不应期内发放高频刺激建立模型。这种选择性自主神经刺激在所有犬的 SVC 诱发了 Rapid Firing 以及 Rapid Firing 介导的房颤。如图 2-6 所示，Rapid Firing 起源于 SVC，Rapid Firing 的最早激动出现于最后一个高频刺激脉冲后的 100ms，排除了 Rapid Firing 由直接刺激 SVC 肌袖而产生的可能性。SVC-Ao GP 消融后，这种 Rapid Firing 和房颤即使应用最大电压的高频刺激也不能被诱发。然而，消融心房表面肺静脉附近的 4 个主要的 GP（ARGP、IRGP、SLGP 和 ILGP）对 SVC 起源的 Rapid Firing 和房颤无效。静脉推注 esmolol（1 mg/kg）后，房颤阈值由用药前的 4.5V 增加到 9.3V（$P<0.05$）。静脉推注 atropine（1 mg）后，所有犬房颤不能被高频刺激诱发（$P<0.05$）。

讨 论

1. 主要发现

以前的研究提示 SVC-Ao GP 是来自于中枢的迷走神经通向心脏的中继站[5]。本实验发现，SVC-Ao GP 在发挥"中继站"作用的同时，还相对选择性地调控 SVC 的电生理性质，支持点有：①刺激 SVC-Ao GP 在 SVC 产生更为明显的电生理改变（ERP 缩短和

WOV 增加);②消融 SVC-Ao GP 仅能显著增加 SVC 的 ERP 和缩小 SVC 的 WOV;③消融 SVC-Ao GP 能显著抑制 SVC 起源的 Rapid Firing,而消融其他 GP 无效。这些现象提示:起源于 SVC 的 Rapid Firing 可能跟 SVC-Ao GP 的激活有关。

2. SVC-Ao GP 与上下游结构的联系

Chiou 等[5]研究发现,消融 SVC-Ao GP 可以抑制颈部迷走神经刺激导致的心房 ERP 的缩短和易颤性的增加,说明大部分通向心脏的外在迷走神经必须经过 SVC-Ao GP,与本研究结果一致。SVC-Ao GP 是心房表面 GP 的上级结构。本研究中,在消融 SVC-Ao GP 后,高电压刺激迷走交感干仍然能轻度减慢心率和抑制房室传导,说明小部分迷走神经纤维可能绕过 SVC-Ao GP 直接与心房表面的内在神经系统相连接,这可能是颈部迷走交感干刺激相对于 SVC-Ao GP 刺激而言,效果更弥散和更均一的重要原因。本研究最重要的发现是,SVC-Ao GP 对于 SVC 的影响具有相对选择性,这可能跟二者的毗邻关系有关。我们推测,SVC-Ao GP 可能通过位于其下游的心房表面 GP 对心房和肺静脉的电生理性质产生间接影响,而可能发出神经纤维对 SVC 进行直接调控(图 2-7)。组织学研究发现了 SVC 肌袖内含有大量的自主神经纤维[14~16],支持这一推测。

3. SVC Firing 的自主神经机制

在以前的研究中[6,7],我们发现了肺静脉起源的 Rapid Firing 是在交感和副交感成分的共同作用下产生的。前者缩短心肌不应期而后者通过增加细胞内的钙离子浓度使早后除极增加,Firing 在心肌不应期缩短的前提下,由早后除极诱发。Marshall 韧带是肺静脉以外的另一个异位激动灶。最新的研究表明,Marshall 韧带起源的 Rapid Firing 亦依赖于交感和副交感的共同激活[12]。本研究中,esmolol 和 atropine 显著抑制或消除 SVC 起源的 Rapid Firing,说明了交感和副交感成分均参与了 SVC 起源的 Rapid Firing 的形成。本研究发现了 SVC-Ao GP 对 SVC 电生理性质的相对选择性,消融 SVC-Ao GP 抑制了 SVC 起源 Rapid Firing,提示起源于 SVC 的 Rapid

Firing 可能与 SVC-Ao GP 的激活有关。

4. 临床意义

临床上，部分阵发性房颤患者的 Rapid Firing 来源于 SVC，通常位于 SVC 的近端后壁[2]。采用射频消融术电隔离 SVC 口部可以中止 Rapid Firing[17,18]，说明 Rapid Firing 的产生和维持需要 SVC 以外的因素支持，电隔离 SVC 口部可能破坏了外界支持因素通向 SVC 的通路。从本研究推测，SVC-Ao GP 很可能就是上述外界支持因素，SVC 口部隔离所取得的成功率可能与破坏 SVC-Ao GP 通向 SVC 的周围的自主神经纤维有关。由此推论，消融 SVC-Ao GP 可能也能消除 SVC 起源的 Rapid Firing，同时可以避免 SVC 隔离带来的损伤膈神经和窦房结的风险。消融心房表面位于肺静脉附近的 GP 对于 SVC 起源的 Rapid Firing 无效。

5. 研究局限性

本研究探讨了 SVC-Ao GP 与上下游结构之间的电生理联系，发现了 SVC-Ao GP 对 SVC 的相对选择性支配，但是这些结论需要进一步的组织学实验加以验证。

在以前的报道中，颈部"迷走交感干"经常被称之为"迷走神经"，实际上后者包含交感成分。对于心房而言，副交感系统兴奋导致 ERP 缩短是最容易观察到的现象，而交感系统兴奋反应过程慢而持久，并且对 ERP 无明显影响。因此本研究中刺激颈部迷走交感干观察到的 ERP 缩短是副交感系统兴奋的结果，我们并没有特意衡量交感兴奋的具体表现。

结　论

本研究表明，SVC-Ao GP 不仅作为外在迷走神经通向心脏内在神经系统的中继站，而且相对选择性地调控 SVC 的电生理性质。消融 SVC-Ao GP 抑制了 SVC 起源 Rapid Firing。这些现象提示起源于 SVC 的 Rapid Firing 可能与 SVC-Ao GP 的激活有关。

表 2-1 SVC-Ao GP 消融前后基础状态下 ERP 和 WOV 的变化

			LA	LAA	LSPV	LIPV	RA	RAA	RSPV	RIPV	SVC
2×TH	ERP	消融前	115±13	120±6	109±14	116±7	118±17	121±7	125±10	119±8	120±17
		消融后	118±11	121±9	110±10	121±9	125±16	120±9	124±13	121±9	139±21 *
	WOV	消融前	3±9	0.4±1	0	0	0	0.3±1	0.2±0.6	0	0
		消融后	3±10	0.8±1	0.2±1	0.2±0.6	0	1.5±2	2±7	1±2	0
10×TH	ERP	消融前	95±10	99±13	81±17	101±12	104±17	103±13	95±11	99±9	101±21
		消融后	99±15	103±12	87±16	103±12	107±14	103±12	99±13	102±12	119±14 *
	WOV	消融前	2±5	2±4	11±13	0.7±2	0.6±2	0.6±1	0.7±3	0	2±3
		消融后	3±7	2±3	10±17	0.8±2	3±8	2±3	0	2±2	0 *

*：$P<0.05$ 指 SVC-Ao GP 消融前后比较,差异有统计学意义。SVC-Ao GP 消融显著延长基础状态下 SVC 的 ERP(2×TH 和 10×TH)和降低 SVC 的房颤诱发窗口(10×TH)。

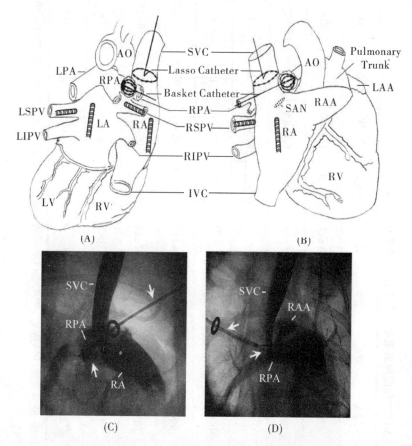

图 2-1 电生理记录导管位置示意图和篮状电极影像学图像
（A）后前位；（B）右侧位。八级电生理记录导管分别缝于左右侧肺静脉（PV）、左右心房和心耳。Lasso 电极导管经颈静脉鞘管送入上腔静脉（SVC）与右房（RA）交界区以上。篮状电极经右肺动脉（RPA）的分支送入 RPA 与 SVC 交界处。（C，D）造影显示篮状电极位于 RPA 主干并与 SVC 相邻。SAN：窦房结；LA：左心房；LV：左心室；RV：右心室；IVC：下腔静脉；RAA：右心耳；LAA：左心耳。

第2章　上腔静脉起源的快速电激动的自主神经机制

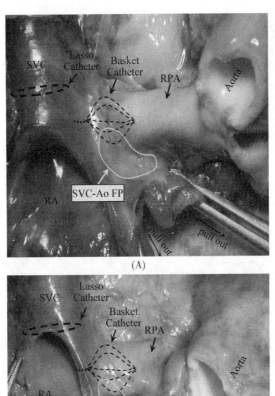

图 2-2　SVC-Ao GP 的部位以及与周围结构的关系

(A) SVC-Ao GP 经篮状电极和刺激/消融笔定位后,取下心脏,除去大部分心房和心室结构,可见 SVC-Ao GP 位于 RPA、SVC 和主动脉根部交界区的脂肪垫(SVC-Ao FP)内。切去主动脉近段以便更好的显示 SVC-Ao GP。(B) 另一条犬,在定位并消融 SVC-Ao GP 后取下心脏,可见消融部位局限。虚线标明 Lasso 电极和篮状电极所在位置。

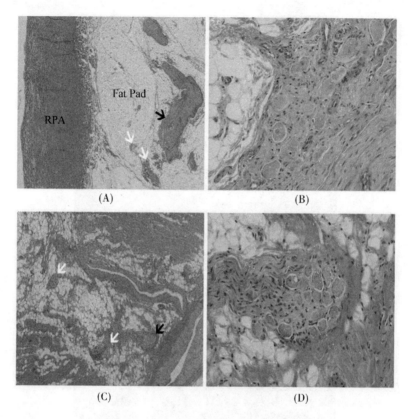

图 2-3　SVC-Ao GP 的组织学染色结果

组织取自图 2-2A 中黄色标记区域。在横切面（A、B）和纵切面（C、D）均能清楚地看到 GP 的分布。黑箭头和白箭头均指向被脂肪组织包裹的 GP。图 B 和 D 分别显示图 A 和 C 中黑箭头标记区域的高倍镜视野，可见 GP 内包含大量神经节细胞。放大倍数分别为（A）2×,（B）20×,（C）4×,（D）20×。

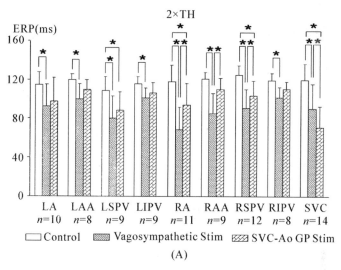

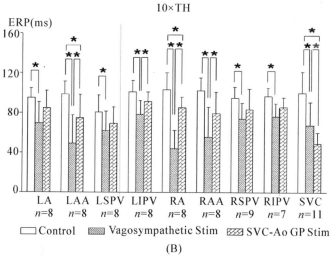

图 2-4 SVC-Ao GP 消融前,刺激 SVC-Ao GP 或同侧迷走交感干对有效不应期(ERP)和心房易颤窗口(WOV)的影响

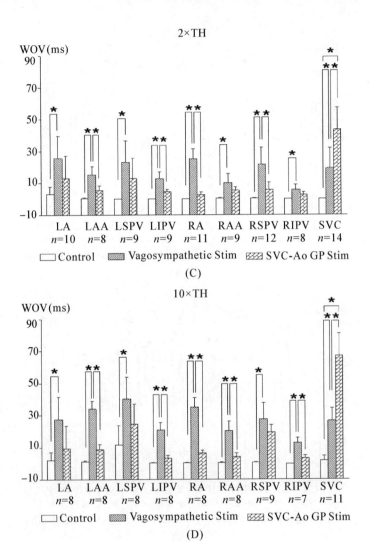

图 2-4 SVC-Ao GP 消融前,刺激 SVC-Ao GP 或同侧迷走交感干对有效
不应期(ERP)和心房易颤窗口(WOV)的影响

(A)2 倍阈值(2×TH)条件下 ERP 的变化;(B)10×TH 条件下 ERP 的变化;
(C)2×TH 条件下 WOV 的变化;(D)10×TH 条件下 WOV 的变化。刺激同
侧迷走交感干使所有部位的 ERP 和 WOV 发生显著变化,然而刺激 SVC-Ao
GP 对 SVC 的影响明显大于其它部位。

第2章 上腔静脉起源的快速电激动的自主神经机制

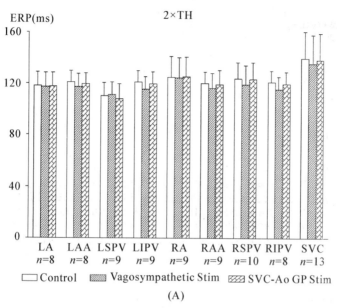

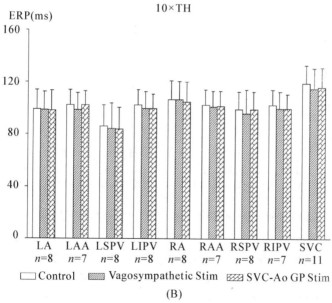

图2-5 SVC-Ao GP 消融后，刺激 SVC-Ao GP 或同侧迷走交感干对 ERP 和 WOV 无明显影响

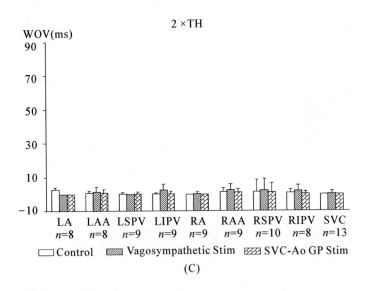

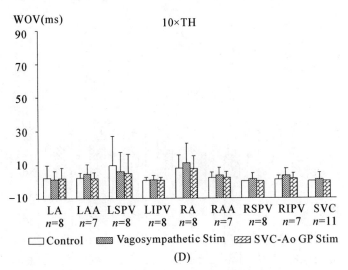

图2-5 SVC-Ao GP 消融后,刺激 SVC-Ao GP 或同侧迷走交感干对 ERP 和 WOV 无明显影响

(A)2×TH 条件下 ERP 的变化;(B) 10×TH 条件下 ERP 的变化;(C) 2×TH 条件下 WOV 的变化;(D) 10×TH 条件下 WOV 的变化。

第2章 上腔静脉起源的快速电激动的自主神经机制

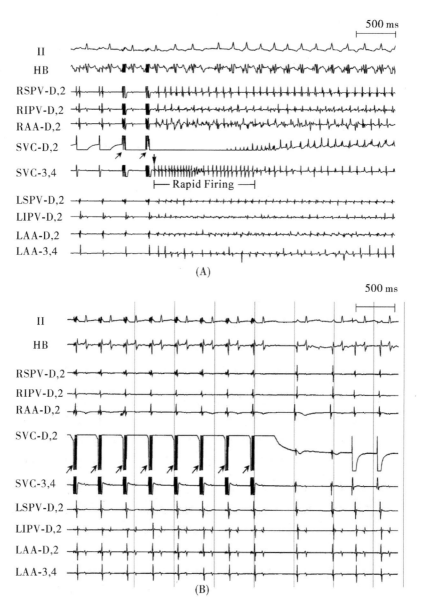

图2-6 消融不同GP后,高频刺激在SVC部位的房颤诱发阈值的变化

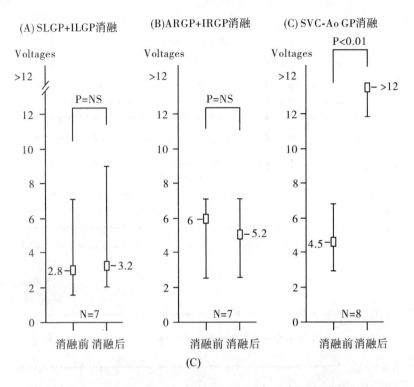

图2-6 消融不同GP后,高频刺激在SVC部位的房颤诱发阈值的变化 (A)心肌不应期内发放的高频刺激(4.5V)诱发Firing和Firing介导的房颤;(B)消融SVC-Ao GP后,最大电压的高频刺激(12V)也不能诱发Firing和房颤;(C)消融心房表面GP(包括SLGP、ILGP、ARGP和IRGP)对SVC的Firing无影响。消融SVC-Ao GP后,在绝大多数犬的SVC不能诱发出Firing和房颤。

第2章 上腔静脉起源的快速电激动的自主神经机制

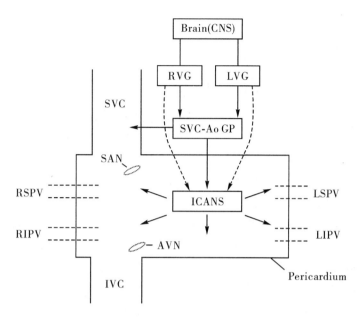

图 2-7 SVC-Ao GP 与上下游结构之间的可能关系。
SVC-Ao GP 是中枢神经系统(CNS)通向心脏的中继站,SVC-Ao GP 对窦房结(SAN)、房室结(AVN)、心房和肺静脉的调控可能是通过心脏内在自主神经系统(ICANS)内的 GP 间接发挥作用。同时,SVC-Ao GP 可能直接发出神经纤维支配 SVC(红色箭头)。RVG:右侧迷走交感干;LVG:左侧迷走交感干;Pericardium:心包。

第3章　心房碎裂电位的自主神经机制

临床上，房颤患者的心房存在不同程度的碎裂电位（CFAE），这是房颤区别于其它类型的房性心律失常的一个重要特征[1,2]。CFAE 的产生被认为与快速电活动在心房内遇到解剖性或功能性传导阻滞有关[3~6]。由此而来的一个重要假说是：CFAE 由规则而快速的心房激动造成，即房颤的驱动因素在向外传导的过程中遇到解剖或功能不应期而发生颤动样传导[4~6]。Nademanee 等[1]倡导了以 CFAE 为消融靶点的手术方式，尽管目前电生理界对这种手术方式的效果尚存在争议[7~9]，但是已有多个临床研究证明，针对 CFAE 的消融术式能根治大部分阵发性房颤[10,11]。Nademanee 等认为[1]，CFAE 所在区域是房颤维持的关键区域，可以作为房颤的消融靶点。非常有趣的是，Nademanee 报道的 CFAE 区域均涵盖 GP 所在部位[12,13]。这一现象提示：心脏内在自主神经系统可能参与了碎裂电位的产生机制和优势分布。

本研究中，我们拟在心耳表面应用 Ach 或在含 GP 的脂肪垫内注入 Ach 造成持续性房颤模型，用傅立叶转换（FFT）软件来定量分析心房碎裂电位的特点和分布，进一步通过 GP 消融来观察破坏心脏内在自主神经系统对心房碎裂电位的影响。

材料和方法

1. 动物模型的制备

正常成年杂种犬共 35 只，体重 20~25kg，以戊巴比妥钠

50mg/kg 麻醉后，气管插管机械通气。分离双侧股动、静脉，分别置入鞘管。右侧股静脉鞘管内送入体温调节仪，使体温维持在 36.5±1.5℃。左侧股静脉用于滴注生理盐水，维持液体平衡。右侧股动脉用于监测动脉血压。左侧股动脉内送入四极标测导管至主动脉根部无冠窦记录 His 电位。分离双侧颈部迷走神经。持续记录肢体导联 ECG。

经左侧第四肋间开胸，剪开心包，暴露心脏（图 3-1）。将八极电生理记录导管分别缝于 LAA、LSPV 和 LIPV，将另一根六级导管（电极间距 2mm-5mm-2mm）横跨 LA 侧壁，远端（LA_{AA}）指向 LAA，近端（LA_{GP}）指向 SLGP。同样，经右侧第四肋间开胸（图 3-1），将八级电生理导管缝于 RAA、RSPV 和 RIPV 表面，将另一根六极导管横跨 RA 前壁，近端（RA_{AA}）和远端（RA_{GP}）分别指向 RAA 和 ARGP。所有电生理信号由巴德电生理记录系统（美国巴德公司生产）记录，滤波设置为 1~1300Hz。

2. 实验设计

实验 1：心耳表面应用 Ach 诱发持续性房颤

实验 1 的目的是在心耳表面应用 Ach 诱发持续快速电激动驱动房颤，观察房颤过程中 CFAE 的分布。如果 CFAE 是由快速电激动向外传导过程中发生颤动样传导造成，那么越靠近心耳的部位其碎裂电位就会越明显。具体方法（图 3-1A 和图 3-1B）是：在 LAA 或 RAA 表面放置一块经 10mmol/L Ach 湿润过的三角形小纱布（表面积约 240mm²）。为了防止 Ach 渗透至心房，在放置纱布前，将一细塑料管（Barrier）横跨于心耳与心房交界处，并在靠近心耳的一侧涂上组织胶防漏。当房颤自发产生或轻触诱发后，在所有导管记录部位同步获取 30s 电图供分析用。移除纱布，冲洗心耳，待血压和心率回到基础水平后，将更高浓度（100mmol/L）的 Ach 纱布重新放置于心耳表面，记录房颤发生后 30s 的电图。

心房 GP 消融方法：GP 的定位和消融采用美国 AtriCure 公司生产的刺激/消融两用笔进行（同本书第 1 章所述）。GP 位于心外膜脂肪垫内。在解剖学基础上，采用快速电刺激对 GP 进行精确定位。快速电刺激时出现心率明显减慢且减慢程度与刺激电压成正比为阳性反应。一旦发现阳性反应，立即由刺激模式转换为消融模式，直接放电消融。GP消融有效的标志是在最强刺激电压(12V)的情况下所有部位的阳性反应消失。

在LAA或RAA表面应用Ach后，消融对应GP(LAA对应SLGP和ILGP，RAA对应ARGP和IRGP)，重复应用Ach，观察GP消融前后心房CFAE的变化。

实验2：脂肪垫内注射Ach诱发持续性房颤

为了进一步验证心脏内在自主神经系统对CFAE的影响，我们通过微注射器将10mmol/L Ach直接注入包含ARGP或SLGP的脂肪垫内(图3-1C和图3-1D)。以前的研究表明[14]，将Ach注入含GP的脂肪垫内，能在肺静脉-心房交界区产生持续(>3min)的快速电激动；而将等量的Ach注入不含GP的脂肪垫，房颤仅能维持数十秒，说明前者持续快速的电激动并非由于注入的Ach对心房肌的直接作用，而是通过兴奋GP导致更为强烈和持久的递质释放造成的。当房颤自发产生或轻触诱发后，在所有导管记录部位同步获取30s电图，然后按照前述方法消融对应GP并观察CFAE的变化。

3. CFAE的特点分析

(1)傅立叶转换(FFT)软件分析

采用常规FFT频谱分析的方法分析碎裂电位的特点(图3-2)。将所有记录电图输入Spike 2软件(英国CED公司)，随机选取30s记录电图中的5s进行分析。分析方法与以前的报道相同[15]，主要参数为：频谱宽度为5~40 Hz，采样点数为4096点，分辨率为0.24Hz。软件自动计算出被测量电图的主频率(dominant frequency, DF)和规则指数(regularity index, RI)。DF反映电图整体快慢程度，DF越高，说明激动越快。RI反映电图的规则程度，越接近0说明电图越紊乱。

(2)手工分析

为了克服软件误识别的弊端，我们手工分析了5s内出现的碎裂电位的总时间，得出碎裂电位的百分比(CFAE%)[16]。根据以往的研究，CFAE 电位定义为大于 3 个波折的电位或持续激动而无等电位线的电位。根据这一定义，转子(rotor)样电图，虽然非常规则但无明显等电位线，因此也归入 CFAE 的范畴(图 3-2)。

(3) 碎裂电位的稳定性分析

为了评价碎裂电位在 30s 内的稳定性，我们分别测量了实验 1 和实验 2 中 CFAE 电图在第 5~10s，第 15~20s，第 25~30s 这三个 5s 内的 DF、RI 和 CFAE%，比较三者在这 3 段时间内的差异。

4. 统计学分析

所有数据采用均数 ± 标准差表示。干预前后(例如应用 Ach 前后，GP 消融前后)各种参数(例如 DF、RI 和 CFAE%)的比较采用配对 T 检验。比较 RA_{AA}、RA_{Mid} 和 RA_{GP} 三者之间以及 LA_{AA}、LA_{Mid}, and LA_{GP} 三者之间 DF、RI 和 CFAE% 的差异采用方差分析。$P<0.05$ 为差异有显著性。

结　　果

碎裂电位的稳定性

实验 1 和实验 2 采用的两种房颤模型中，在第 5~10s、第 15~20s、第 25~30s 这三个 5s 内的 DF、RI 和 CFAE% 并无显著差异，说明至少在 30s 记录时间内，各部位的 CFAE 电图是稳定的(图 3-3)。

实验 1：在 LAA 或 RAA 表面应用 Ach 时，刺激 ARGP 或 SLGP 使心率降低 50% 所需要的电压由刺激前的 2 ± 1.1 V 降低至 1.2 ± 1.1 V($N=11$, $P<0.05$)，诱发房颤所需要的电压由刺激前的 7 ± 3.8 V 降低至 2.8 ± 1.6 V($N=13$, $P<0.05$)。以左侧为例(图 3-1B)，LAA 记录到 rotor 样快速而规则的电图，房颤由 LAA 驱动；而在 LA 和左侧肺静脉部位记录到不同程度的 CFAE。含最高 DF、RI 和 CFAE% 的部位总是 LAA，然而，有趣的是：靠近 LAA 的部位(即 LA_{AA})其碎裂电位的快慢程度和紊乱程度均显著低

于靠近SLGP的部位(即LA$_{GP}$)(图3-4)。DF、RI和CFAE%均出现与颤动样传导相反的梯度：越靠近LAA的部位，DF和CFAE%越低，RI越高；越靠近GP的部位，DF和CFAE%越高，RI越低(图3-5)。除LAA外，最高的DF和CFAE%总是位于靠近SLGP的位置，即LA$_{GP}$或LSPV。当把Ach浓度由10mmol/L增加至100mmol/L时，绝大多数部位的DF和CFAE%均升高而RI降低，但三者在心房分布的梯度依然存在(表3-1，图3-5)。在RAA应用Ach时出现类似现象(图3-4、图3-5和表3-2)。

消融左侧或右侧GP后，将Ach分别重新应用于LAA或RAA表面，心耳依然能诱发出Rotor样电激动，但心耳以外部位的CFAE明显减少或消失，DF和CFAE%降低而RI升高，心房CFAE的分布梯度消失(图3-4，图3-5)。即使Ach由10mmol/L增加至100mmol/L，也仅能增加心耳的DF值，对其它部位的CFAE无明显影响(表3-1和表3-2)。

实验2：当将10mmol/L Ach注入ARGP或SLGP后，窦性心率显著减慢。房颤发生后，靠近ARGP(RA$_{GP}$或RSPV)或SLGP(LA$_{GP}$或LSPV)部位的CFAE最为显著(图3-6)，相同的DF、RI和CFAE%梯度在心房再次出现(图3-7)。

GP消融过程中，心房的CFAE逐渐减少并最终消失(图3-6)。进行了ARGP和IRGP消融的12条犬中的10条(10/12)和进行了SLGP和ILGP消融的全部13条犬(13/13)在GP消融过程中，房颤终止并且难以被再次诱发。由于房颤在消融过程中终止并且不易被再次诱发，DF、RI和CFAE%在GP消融后不能获得。

讨 论

1. 主要发现

本研究采用的两种不同的房颤模型中，心房的CFAE出现了相同的梯度：DF和CFAE%从GP向远处逐渐降低，RI从GP向远处逐渐升高。GP消融后CFAE显著减少或消失，并且CFAE梯度消失。这些现象表明，以 GP 为核心的心脏内在自主神经系统，在 CFAE 发生机制中发挥了重要作用。

2. 心脏内在自主神经系统和 CFAE 的关系

在实验 1 中，靠近心耳的部位（LA_{AA} 或 RA_{AA}）相对于靠近 GP 的部位（LA_{GP} 或 RA_{GP}）并未出现 CFAE 分布上的优势，至少说明在本模型中，颤动样传导并没有在 CFAE 的产生和分布中起主要作用。以前的研究发现[17]，心房有效不应期（ERP）和房颤诱发窗口（WOV）同样存在着从 GP 向周围逐渐变化的梯度：越靠近 GP 的部位，ERP 越短，WOV 越宽。这种 ERP 和 WOV 变化的梯度以及本研究中 DF、RI 和 CFAE% 的梯度可能与自主神经纤维密度和神经递质浓度的梯度有关[18~21]。本研究中，激活 GP 或消融 GP 后，这些 CFAE 梯度相应出现或消失，说明了以 GP 为核心的心脏内在自主神经系统的激活可能是 CFAE 产生的重要机制。实验 1 中，心耳表面应用 Ach 后，GP 对电刺激的反应明显增强；实验 2 中，将 Ach 注入 GP 后，心率明显降低，这些现象是 GP 被激活的证据。我们推测：GP 激活随之释放的大量神经递质（包括交感神经递质和副交感神经递质）可能参与了 CFAE 的形成和分布。

3. 心-心反射和房颤

传统观念认为，GP 只是中枢神经系统通向心脏的中继站。Ardell 等[22]通过系统的研究发现，GP 不仅仅是上传下达的中继站，而是具有独立调控能力的"微脑"系统，是心脏局部神经反射网络中的核心。GP 内含有大量神经元，这些神经元发出树突和轴突至临近的肺静脉和心房以及远处的心耳。我们认为：心耳局部应用 Ach 时，分布在心耳表面的传入纤维将刺激信号传回至 GP，GP 激活后又通过传出纤维沿着轴突的分布释放大量的神经递质（ACH 和 NE）诱发了 CFAE。越靠近 GP 的部位，神经纤维密度越大，因此 CFAE 也越明显。心脏局部神经兴奋能在短时间内通过快速的神经传导使 GP 高度兴奋，我们称这种神经传导模式为心-心反射（图 3-8）。本研究中，在心耳表面应用 Ach 时，GP 对电刺激的反应明显增强是 GP 被激活的证据。GP 消融后，在心耳表面再次应用 Ach 时，由于神经传导网络被破坏，仅在心耳产生微弱的局部反应，心耳以外的 CFAE 明显减少并且梯度消失，支持 GP 在心-心反射中发挥核心作用。

4. 临床意义

Nademanee 等[1]的临床研究发现，CFAE 易分布在某些区域，例如肺静脉与心房交界区、房间隔等，这些部位恰好包含 GP 所在部位[12,13]。在报道中，作者推测以 CFAE 为靶点的消融术式所取得的效果可能部分与破坏 GP 有关。这一推测在本研究中得到支持，自主神经系统的激活和神经递质的释放可能是 CFAE 的产生和分布的重要机制。临床上，CFAE 消融的问题在于：由于 CFAE 电位在心房的分布广泛并且不稳定，因此消融过程中不可避免地损伤无辜的心房肌，可能影响术后心房功能的恢复。相对于 CFAE 消融，GP 消融有可能达到既消除房颤，又减少心房损伤的目的，这一推论需要进一步的临床研究加以检验。

5. 研究局限性

本研究中，我们在心耳表面应用 10mmol/L 或 100mmol/L 的 Ach 诱发持续性 AF（>3 分钟），存在这样的可能性：少量 Ach 渗透入血液循环中，影响实验结果。为验证这种可能性，我们将少量 Ach 直接注入心耳腔内，结果心脏出现强烈的类迷走反应，但 AF 仅能维持 20s 左右，说明注入的 Ach 被迅速代谢[24]。实际上，即使少量的 Ach 进入血液循环，发生房颤时，CFAE 应当是在整个心房弥漫性分布而不会出现本研究中观察到的梯度。

我们并没有设计专门的实验排除中枢神经系统的影响，但是尝试了剪断 2 条犬颈部的迷走神经和消融星状神经节，从而切断中枢神经系统跟心脏的联系，但实验结果与保留中枢神经系统联系并无明显区别。

结　　论

本研究中，我们在构建的两种房颤模型中观察到 CFAE 从 GP 到外周递减分布的梯度。消融 GP 后，CFAE 明显减少或消失，并且分布梯度消失，说明了心脏内在自主神经系统的激活是 CFAE 产生的重要机制，同时提示了以 GP 为核心的心-心反射在调控心脏各种电生理性质中发挥了重要作用。

表 3-1 实验 1 中 GP 消融前后左心耳应用 Ach 后 CFAE 的分布

			LAA	LA_{AA}	LA_{MID}	LA_{GP}	LSPV-D2	LIPV-D2
10 mmol/L Ach on LAA	DF (Hz)	Before ablation	22±9	11±4	12±3	13±5	13±87	12±5
		After ablation	18±8	8±2	9±1	9±1	10±3	9±1
		P_1 Value	0.3	<0.05	<0.05	<0.05	0.05	<0.05
	RI	Before ablation	0.4±0.2	0.4±0.07	0.4±0.1	0.3±0.1	0.4±0.1	0.4±0.08
		After ablation	0.5±0.2	0.5±0.2	0.5±0.12	0.5±0.2	0.6±0.1	0.6±0.1
		P_2 Value	0.2	0.2	<0.05	<0.01	<0.01	<0.01
	CFAE% (%)	Before ablation	88±20	48±16	65±12	81±17	60±30	25±15
		After ablation	88±21	20±22	19±23	25±24	6±10	3±7
		P_3 Value	0.85	<0.01	<0.01	<0.01	<0.01	<0.01
100 mmol/L Ach on LAA	DF (Hz)	Before ablation	28±8##	13±5#	16±6##	19±7#	20±11#	13±6
		After ablation	22±8	10±2	10±2	9±1	9±1	11±5
		P_1 Value	<0.05	0.05	<0.01	<0.01	<0.01	<0.05
	RI	Before ablation	0.5±0.1	0.4±0.05##	0.3±0.1#	0.3±0.1	0.3±0.1#	0.3±0.1
		After ablation	0.6±0.2	0.5±0.2	0.5±0.2	0.5±0.2	0.7±0.1	0.7±0.1
		P_2 Value	0.2	<0.05	<0.01	<0.01	<0.01	<0.01
	CFAE% (%)	Before ablation	99±1	75±9##	85±6##	98±5##	74±34#	34±25
		After ablation	93±10	28±27	22±24	26±23	7±12	3±8
		P_3 Value	0.08	<0.01	<0.01	<0.01	<0.01	<0.01

P1,P2,P3 分别指消融前后 DF、RI 和 CFAE% 的差异的 P 值,#和## 分别指 10mmol/L 和 100mmol/L 相比 $P<0.05$ 和 $P<0.01$

表 3-2 实验 1 中 GP 消融前后右心耳应用 Ach 后 CFAE 的分布

			RAA	RA$_{AA}$	RA$_{MID}$	RA$_{GP}$	RSPV-D2	RIPV-D2
10 mmol/L Ach on RAA	DF (Hz)	Before ablation	23±7	9±1	10±3	11±3	9±0.8	9±2
		After ablation	15±6	8±1	8±2	8±1	8±0.8	8±1
		P$_1$	<0.01	0.06	<0.05	<0.01	<0.05	0.1
	RI	Before ablation	0.4±0.1	0.4±0.1	0.3±0.09	0.3±0.08	0.4±0.2	0.4±0.1
		After ablation	0.5±0.2	0.5±0.2	0.5±0.1	0.6±0.2	0.7±0.2	0.7±0.2
		P$_2$	<0.05	0.06	<0.01	<0.01	<0.01	<0.01
	CFAE% (%)	Before ablation	86±17	34±24	39±18	63±27	40±28	32±24
		After ablation	74±35	14±11	13±11	23±16	3±6	5±6
		P$_3$	0.2	<0.01	<0.01	<0.01	<0.01	<0.01
100 mmol/L Ach on RAA	DF (Hz)	Before ablation	30±7##	10±1##	11±3##	14±4##	10±3#	12±6
		After ablation	25±5##	8±1	8±2	9±2	8±1	8±1
		P$_1$	0.06	<0.01	<0.01	<0.01	<0.05	<0.05
	RI	Before ablation	0.4±0.2	0.3±0.1##	0.3±0.09##	0.2±0.05##	0.4±0.2	0.4±0.2
		After ablation	0.7±0.2#	0.5±0.2	0.5±0.1	0.5±0.2	0.7±0.2	0.7±0.2
		P$_2$	<0.05	<0.01	<0.01	<0.01	<0.01	<0.01
	CFAE% (%)	Before ablation	96±7#	74±21##	81±20##	93±9##	57±28##	47±29#
		After ablation	98±6	15±12	16±13	27±20	2±4	2±4
		P$_3$	0.34	<0.01	<0.01	<0.01	<0.01	<0.01

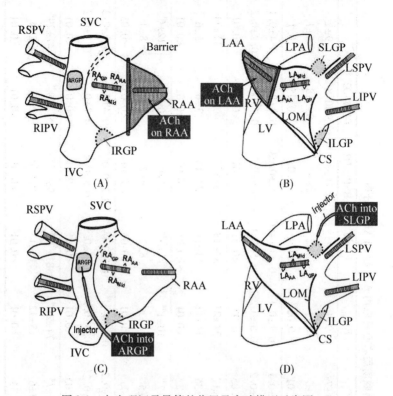

图 3-1　电生理记录导管的位置及实验模型示意图

（A）实验 1 中右侧开胸。八极电生理记录导管（电极间距 2mm）分别缝于 RAA、RSPV 和 RIPV，将另一根六级（电极间距 2mm-5mm-2mm）横跨右心房，近端电极对（RA_{AA}）指向 RAA，远端电极对（RA_{GP}）指向 ARGP，中间电极对（RA_{Mid}）记录 RA 中部电位。在 RAA 放置一块三角形的经 Ach 溶液湿润过的纱布，将一细塑料管（Barrier）横跨于心耳与心房交界处阻止 Ach 渗漏；（B）实验 1 中左侧开胸，导管放置方法及实验模型与右侧类似；（C）导管记录方法与图 A 相同。将 10mmol/L Ach 经微注射器注入包含 ARGP 的脂肪垫内；（D）导管记录方法与图 B 相同。将 10mmol/L Ach 注入包含 SLGP 的脂肪垫内。

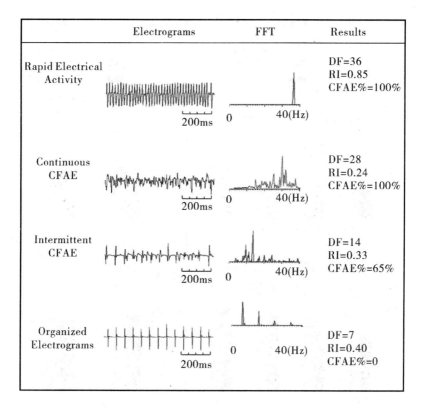

图 3-2　4 种不同类型的电图采用 FFT 软件分析和手工分析的实例
第一种快速规则的 Rotor 样电图由于无等电位线，其 CFAE% 计为 100%。

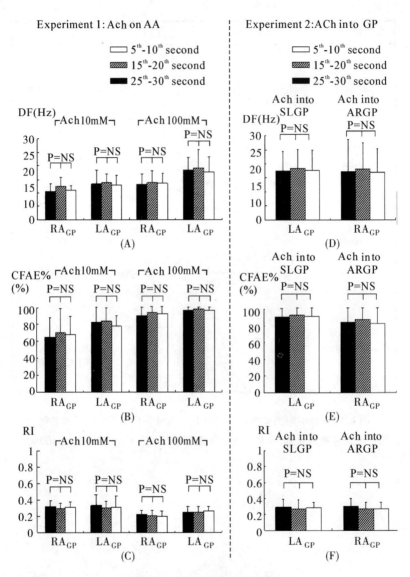

图 3-3 CFAE 的稳定性分析

以靠近 GP 的位点（RA_{GP} 和 LA_{GP}）为例，分析 CFAE 在两个实验中的稳定性，结果显示 CFAE 的 DF、RI 和 CFAE% 在第 5~10s、第 15~20s 和第 25~30s 三个时间段内无明显差异。

第3章 心房碎裂电位的自主神经机制

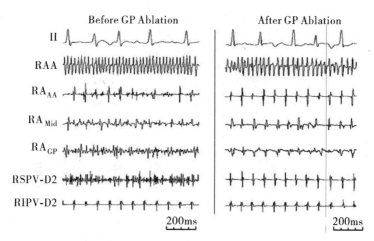

(A) Right Thoracotomy Approach

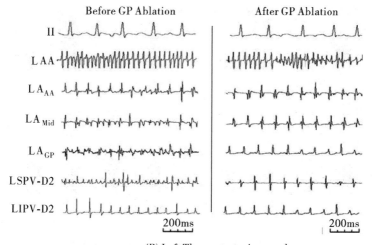

(B) Left Thoracotomy Approach

图 3-4　实验 1 中，GP 消融前后各部位 CFAE 的变化

(A) 右侧开胸，将 10mmol/L Ach 应用于右心耳诱发出 Rotor 样快速规则的电图，然而心房上靠近心耳的部位（RA_{AA}）其 CFAE 不如靠近 ARGP 的部位（RA_{GP}）明显，与颤动样传导理论相反。GP 消融后，CFAE 明显减少并且分布梯度消失。(B) 左侧开胸，将 10mmol/L Ach 应用于左心耳，结果与右侧类似。

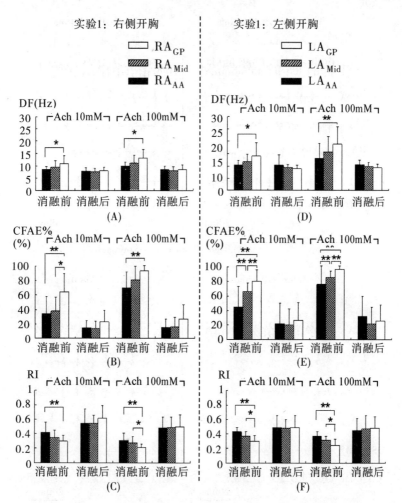

图 3-5 实验 1 中，GP 消融前后 CFAE 的分布梯度

GP 消融前，无论是在心耳应用 10mmol/L 还是 100mmol/L Ach，越靠近心耳的部位，DF 和 CFAE% 越低，RI 越高；越靠近 GP 的部位，DF 和 CFAE% 越高，RI 越低。GP 消融后，CFAE 明显减少，其分布梯度消失。

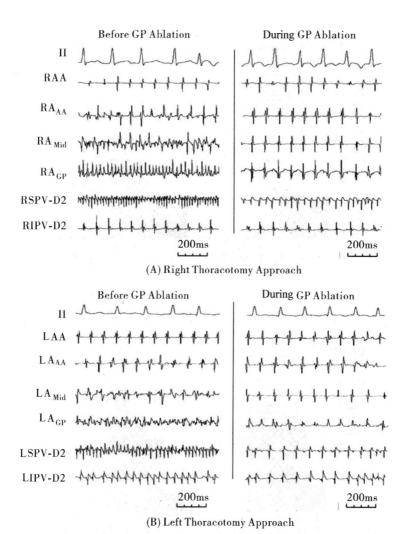

图 3-6 实验 2 中，Ach 注入 GP 后 CFAE 的分布和消融过程中的变化 当 10mmol/L Ach 注入 ARGP 或 SLGP 后，GP 周围出现 Firing，越靠近 GP，CFAE 越显著；在 GP 消融过程中，CFAE 慢慢减少直至房颤中止。

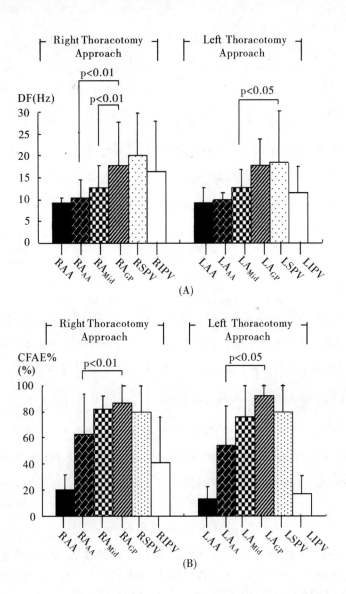

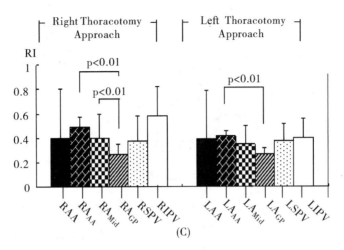

图 3-7 实验 2 中,Ach 注入 GP 后 CFAE 的分布和梯度

RA_{GP}、RA_{Mid} 和 RA_{AA} 三者之间以及 LA_{GP}、LA_{Mid} 和 LA_{AA} 三者之间 CFAE 的分布梯度与图 3-5 类似,越靠近 GP 的部位,CFAE 越显著。

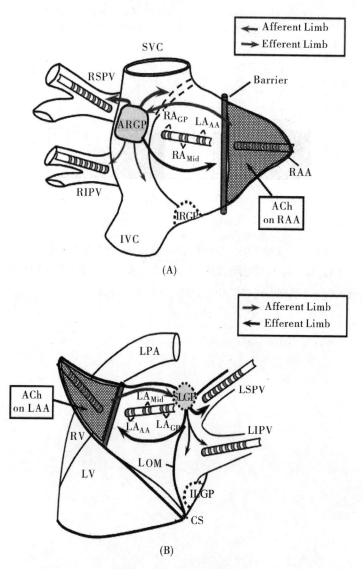

图 3-8 心-心反射示意图

见文中详述。Afferent Limb 为传入神经纤维，Efferent Limb 为传出神经纤维。

第4章　房颤致房颤现象的自主神经机制

1995年，Wijffels等[1]发现对山羊的心房进行慢性快速起搏可以导致心房有效不应期的缩短和房颤维持时间的延长。心房起搏时间越长，AF持续时间也越长。他们称这种现象为"房颤致房颤"。这一现象引起了临床医生的重视，因为"房颤致房颤"可以用来解释为什么频繁发作的阵发性房颤常常转化为持续性甚至永久性房颤。近十年来，大量的研究发现，"房颤致房颤"的机制可能跟长期快速起搏造成的心房结构重构和电重构有关[2,3]。房颤持续时间越长，心房重构越显著。近来，基础研究表明，以GP为核心的心脏内在自主神经系统(ICANS)在房颤的诱发和维持中发挥了重要作用[4~11]。本研究中，我们构建了犬心房快速起搏模型，在起搏前和起搏后消融位于心房外膜脂肪垫内的GP，探讨心脏内在自主神经系统在心房急性电重构中的作用。

材料和方法

1. 动物模型的制备

正常成年杂种犬共18只，体重20~25kg，以戊巴比妥钠50mg/kg麻醉后，气管插管机械通气。分离双侧股动、静脉，分别置入鞘管。右侧股静脉鞘管内送入体温调节仪，使体温维持在36.5±1.5℃。左侧股静脉用于滴注生理盐水，维持液体平衡。右侧股动脉用于监测动脉血压。左侧股动脉内送入四极标测导管至主动脉根部无冠窦记录His电位。持续记录肢体导联ECG。

经左侧第四肋间开胸，剪开心包，暴露心脏。将多极电生理记录导管分别缝于 LAA、LA、LSPV 和 LIPV 表面（图 4-1A）。同样，经右侧第四肋间开胸，将导管缝于 RAA、RA、RSPV 和 RIPV 表面（图 4-1B）。所有电生理信号由巴德电生理记录系统（美国巴德公司生产）记录和分析，滤波设置在 30~250Hz。

2. 快速起搏与程控电刺激

在 LAA 发放总计 6h 的快速起搏，起搏频率为 1200bpm，电压为 2 倍阈值，脉宽为 1ms。6h 起搏过程中，每隔 1h 起搏暂停以便进行 ERP 和房颤诱发性的测量。程控电刺激由程控刺激仪发放（Medtronic Inc，USA）。ERP 采用 S1S2 递减的方法测量：S1－S1＝330ms，S1∶S2＝8∶1，刺激电压分别采用 2 倍起搏阈值（2×TH）和 10 倍起搏阈值（10×TH）。S1S2 从 150ms 递减，步长 10ms，当遇到不应期时，从上一个 S1S2 间期起，步长减为 1ms。在 7 个部位（LSPV、LIPV、LA、RSPV、RIPV、RA 和 RAA）分别测量 2×TH 和 10×TH 下的 ERP。ERP 离散度定义为以上 7 个部位的 ERP 的标准差与均数之商[12]。

房颤的诱发性采用心房易颤窗口（WOV）的大小来衡量[5]。房颤定义为持续 5s 以上的快速而不规则心房激动（>500bpm）伴不规则房室传导。在 ERP 测量过程中，如果 S1S2 刺激诱发了房颤，那么紧接着测量能诱发房颤的最长和最短 S1S2 间期，二者之差为房颤的易颤窗口。ΣWOV 定义为在所有测量部位 2×TH 和 10×TH 下的 WOV 的总和，用来评价整条犬诱发房颤的难易程度。若房颤不能被诱发，WOV 计为 0。在大多数情况下，ERP 和 WOV 的测量在 15min 内完成。

3. GP 消融

GP 的消融方法同前所述。在解剖学基础上，采用快速电刺激（20Hz，0.1ms，1~12V）对 GP 进行精确定位。快速电刺激时出现心率明显减慢且减慢程度与刺激电压成正比为阳性反应。刺激和消融均采用美国 AtriCure 生产的刺激/消融两用笔进行。一旦发现阳性反应，立即由刺激模式转换到消融模式，直接放电消融。GP消融有效的标志是在最强电压(12V)刺激情况下所有阳性反应消失。ARGP、IRGP、SLGP、ILGP 以及 Marshall 韧带(LOM)内的 GP 均采用以上方法消融。消融后 GP 周边心房电位的形态和幅度没有发生明显变化，说明 GP 消融对周边心房肌的损伤轻微(见本书第一部分图1-7)。

4. 自主神经阻滞剂的应用

为了进一步评价自主神经系统的作用，我们应用阿托品和普萘洛尔同时阻滞副交感神经系统和交感神经系统。这两种药物按照 Wijffels 等[13]报道的方法给药。硫酸阿托品溶液(Sigma-Aldrich Inc, USA)1.0 mg/kg 和盐酸普萘洛尔溶液 0.6 mg/kg(Sigma-Aldrich Inc, USA)分别在10min内经股静脉缓慢推注。

5. 实验分组和设计

第一组($N=7$)：6h 快速起搏后立即进行 GP (ARGP + IRGP + SLGP + ILGP + LOM)消融；

第二组($N=7$)：GP(ARGP + IRGP + SLGP + ILGP + LOM)消融后立即进行6h 快速起搏；

第三组($N=4$)：自主神经阻滞剂应用后立即进行6h 快速起搏。

在总共6h 快速起搏过程中每隔1h 测量 LSPV、LIPV、LA、RSPV、RIPV、RA 和 RAA 在 $2 \times TH$ 和 $10 \times TH$ 下的 ERP 和 WOV，计算出 ERP 离散度和 ΣWOV。在 GP 消融后和应用自主神经阻滞剂后立即重复测量 ERP 和 WOV。

6. 统计学处理

所有数据采用均数±标准差表示。配对 T 检验用来比较 GP 消融后 ERP 和 WOV 的变化。重复测量的方差分析用来比较不同起搏时间段的 ERP 和 WOV 的变化。采用 LSD 检验进一步比较不同起搏时间段的 ERP 和 WOV 与起搏前基础状态下的差异。

结　　果

在整个实验过程中，所有犬的收缩压和舒张压平稳，在 6h 起搏过程中，没有心衰的证据。

1. ERP 和 WOV

第 1 组（6h 快速起搏后进行 GP 消融，图 4-2）：所有部位的 ERP（$2 \times TH$ 和 $10 \times TH$）在快速起搏后的前两小时显著缩短，但是更长时间的起搏（第 3~6h）不能使 ERP 进一步缩短。然而在 6h 的起搏过程中，ΣWOV 逐渐增加。以 LSPV 为例，2h 起搏后，ERP（$2 \times TH$）从基础状态下的 125 ± 19ms 缩短至 96 ± 14ms，但从第 3h 到第 6h 末，ERP（$2 \times TH$）维持在 90~100ms 之间。WOV 从基础状态下的 5ms 逐渐增加至第 6h 末的 319ms。GP（ARGP + IRGP + SLGP + ILGP + LOM）消融后，所有部位的 ERP 恢复到基础水平，并且未能在任何部位诱发房颤（WOV = 0）。

第 2 组（GP 消融后进行 6h 快速起搏，图 4-3）：GP 消融后，6h 的快速起搏不能缩短任何部位的 ERP。7 条犬中的 6 条不能诱发房颤，而另一条犬仅在 $10 \times TH$ 下在第 3h 诱发房颤（WOV 仅为 10ms），而在第 4~6h 未能诱发房颤。

第 3 组（应用自主神经阻滞剂后进行 6h 快速起搏，图 4-4）：与第 2 组结果类似，应用自主神经阻滞剂后，6h 的快速起搏不能缩短任何部位的 ERP，并且也不能在任何部位诱发房颤。

2. ERP 离散度

第 1 组（表 4-1）：ERP 离散度在起搏后的第 1h 显著增加，但是随后更长时间的起搏并没有导致其进一步增加。GP 消融后，ERP 离散度缩短，但是没有达到统计学差异（$2 \times TH$：$P = 0.08$；$10 \times TH$：$P = 0.10$）。

第 2 组（表 4-2）：GP 消融后，6h 快速心耳起搏没有增加 ERP 离散度。

第 3 组的结果与第 2 组相似。

讨 论

1. 主要发现

本研究中，我们利用快速左心耳起搏获得心房急性电重构模型，表现为 ERP 的缩短、ERP 离散度的增加和 WOV 的不断增宽。消融心房上 4 个主要的 GP 以及 LOM 逆转了 ERP 的缩短，并且在所有测量部位消除了房颤的诱发能力。此外，在预先进行 GP 消融或应用自主神经阻滞剂后，6h 快速起搏不能缩短任何部位的 ERP，也不能诱发房颤（第 2 组：6/7；第 3 组：4/4）。这些现象说明了破坏 ICANS 能逆转和阻止快速心耳起搏造成的急性心房电重构，说明了以 GP 为核心的 ICANS 在急性心房电重构中发挥了重要的作用。

2. "房颤致房颤"的机制

自从 Moe[14] 提出多发子波折返学说以来，房颤的机制被认为与心房内一定数量的折返子波随机游走和碰撞有关。这一理论尤其适用于解释"房颤致房颤"这一电生理现象。但是近 10 年的临床研究发现[15,16]，大多数阵发性或持续性房颤由肺静脉内的局灶性快速电激动驱动。在经典的"房颤致房颤"的动物模型中，Morillo 等[17] 发现左房后壁临近肺静脉-心房交界区存在持续快速电激动，很可能是驱动房颤的关键因素。在类似的动物模型中，Zhou 等[18] 和 Chou 等[19] 应用高精度光学标测方法观察到起源于肺静脉的局灶性快速电活动与房颤的维持相关。这些研究说明，多发子波折返和局灶驱动同时参与了"房颤致房颤"的机制。

已有的研究发现[4,10,11]，驱动房颤的局灶性快速电激动可以通过刺激心脏内在自主神经系统诱发，而破坏心脏内在自主神经系统后不能再诱发。在心脏内在自主神经系统中，GP 包含了最大数量的神经成分，既含副交感成分也含交感成分[20]，是这一系统的核心。本研究中我们推测，GP消融抑制了局灶性快速电激动的产生，并且阻止了所有心房部位ERP的缩短和ERP离散度的增加，使整个心房的异质性缩小，降低了多发子波折返的可能性。也就是说，本试验中GP消融同时抑制了局灶性电活动和多发子波折返，从而抑制了房颤的发生。

3. 急性电重构的机制

在长期慢性心房起搏的模型中，心房结构重构和电重构被认为是导致房颤发生和维持的两个关键因素[3,16,21]，结构重构同时也是导致电重构的重要原因。快速起搏诱导的结构重构不能解释本研究的结果，原因是结构重构常常需要至少持续数天的快速起搏。以前的研究认为心房电重构与快速起搏造成的钙超载有关。钙超载可以导致心房离子通道的改变，尤其是L型钙电流的下调，紧接着导致心房动作电位时程和ERP的缩短[2,3,22,23]。单纯的钙超载和钙电流的改变也不足以解释本研究中的急性电重构现象，因为抑制ICANS（第2组和第3组）阻止了相同起搏方法造成的急性电重构的发生。有学者认为ERP离散度的增加是快速心房起搏导致电重构的另外一个原因[12]。本研究中，我们观察到起搏过程中ERP离散度增加的趋势，但被GP消融所消除（第1组）。在第2组中，GP消融阻止了ERP离散度的增加。这些研究结果提示GP消融抑制房颤的效果至少部分与降低ERP离散度有关。

Wijffels等[1]在早期的研究中推测，心脏自主神经的活性或敏感性改变可能是快速心房起搏导致电重构的一个重要机制。他们为了验证这个推测，在快速起搏山羊的心房数周后，应用自主神经阻滞剂（阿托品和普萘洛尔，剂量与给药方法与本实验相同）结果仅能部分逆转ERP的缩短[13]。值得注意的是，自主神经阻滞剂是在长期快速起搏诱发的房颤持续1~3d后应用。Wijffels等的研究结果与本实验结果之间的差异可以用短期（6h）快速起搏和长期（数周）快速起搏造成心电房重构的机制不同来解释。离子通道蛋白表达的改变和心房结构的改变可能是慢性起搏导致心房电重构的主要原因，然而心脏自主神经系统在短期快速起搏导致的急性心房电重构中发挥了关键作用。

本实验结果说明 ICANS 参与了快速起搏导致急性心房电重构的机制。我们推测 ERP 的缩短至少部分与 ICANS 的激活有关。破坏 ICANS 不仅直接延长了 ERP，而且抑制了自主神经对快速心房起搏的反应。在第 2 组和第 3 组动物中，抑制 ICANS 阻止房颤的机制可能包括：①消融 GP 或应用自主神经阻滞剂导致 ERP 延长和离散度降低，保护了大部分心房肌。也就是说，多发子波在大部分心房肌上不能随机快速扩散，心房不能提供容纳多发子波折返的空间。②Jayachandran 等[24]曾经观察到快速起搏可以导致心房自主神经系统分布和活性的不均一性增加，他们称为"自主神经重构"。自主神经重构促进了房颤的发生。本研究中，破坏 ICANS 可能抑制了快速起搏导致的自主神经重构的发生。③有研究发现[25,26]，某些受自主神经调控的离子通道（例如 $I_{K,ACH}$ 的亚型 I_{KH}）在快速起搏诱发的心房电重构中发挥了重要作用，这些通道可能因为破坏 ICANS 而被抑制。

4. 临床意义

本研究提示 GP 消融能逆转和阻止快速心房起搏导致的急性电重构，这可能是 GP 消融对持续性房颤患者亦有效的重要原因。ICANS 可能在阵发性房颤进展为持续性房颤的过程中发挥了重要作用，破坏 ICANS 可能会阻止这一过程。此外，在心房存在轻度或中度电重构的房颤患者，GP 消融可能会逆转电重构。

目前有观点认为：仅"迷走性房颤"与自主神经有关，GP 消融可能仅在这一类房颤中有效。本研究表明，GP 消融能逆转和阻止经典的"房颤致房颤"现象，提示 GP 不仅仅跟迷走性房颤有关，而且可能是大多数房颤的共同机制之一。

5. 研究的局限性

首先，本研究强烈提示 ICANS 可能与快速心房起搏导致的急性电重构有关，但是需要进一步研究提供直接的证据：包括自主神经激活和病理解剖学的改变。

其次，在第 1 组实验中，在 GP 的定位和消融过程中，由于起搏的中止，心房逆重构（ERP 和 WOV 的恢复）可能发生，因此放大了 GP 消融的效果。为了验证这个可能性，我们进行了对照实验（图4-5）。将 1 条犬按相同方法进行快速起搏 6h 后，不消融 GP 而是观察空白期 ERP 和 ΣWOV 的改变。结果发现，相对于起搏前的基础状态，ERP 即使在起搏中止后的 1h 内仍然较短，ΣWOV 在起搏中止后的 1h 仍维持在 116ms。这说明，相对于 GP 定位和消融所消耗的时间（<15 分钟），心房逆重构是导致 GP 消融后 ERP 和 WOV 改变的次要因素。

最后，ICANS 在长期慢性起搏造成的慢性电重构中的作用有待进一步验证。

结　　论

破坏 ICANS 能逆转和阻止快速心耳起搏造成的急性电重构，某些在急性电重构中发挥重要作用的机制可能被破坏 ICANS 所改变。ICANS 的激活本身可能是导致急性电重构的一个重要原因。本研究提示 ICANS 至少在"房颤致房颤"的急性期发挥了重要作用。

表 4-1　　第 1 组中 GP 消融前后 ERP 离散度的变化

	Baseline	1st hour pacing	2nd hour pacing	3rd hour pacing	4th hour pacing	5th hour pacing	6th hour pacing	GP ablation
2×TH	0.08±0.05	0.11±0.04	0.11±0.05	0.1±0.03	0.12±0.05	0.11±0.06	0.13±0.05	0.06±0.02
10×TH	0.17±0.06	0.26±0.09	0.21±0.06	0.23±0.15	0.22±0.1	0.19±0.07	0.23±0.05	0.13±0.04

ERP 离散度定义为以上 7 个部位（LSPV，LIPV，LA，RSPV，RIPV，RA and RAA）的 ERP 的标准差与均数之商。

表 4-2　　第 2 组中 GP 消融后 ERP 离散度的变化

	GP ablation	1st hour pacing	2nd hour pacing	3rd hour pacing	4th hour pacing	5th hour pacing	6th hour pacing
2×TH	0.11±0.05	0.12±0.05	0.12±0.04	0.12±0.04	0.11±0.03	0.11±0.04	0.11±0.02
10×TH	0.13±0.02	0.15±0.03	0.13±0.01	0.14±0.03	0.12±0.02	0.12±0.04	0.11±0.03

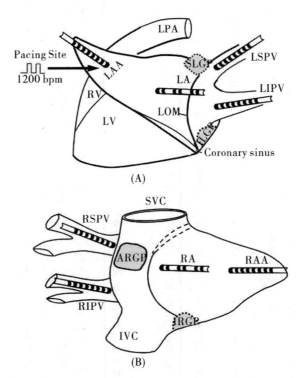

图 4-1　导管记录部位及实验模型

快速左心耳起搏的频率为 1200bpm，起搏电压为 2 倍阈电压。

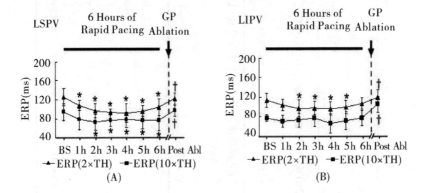

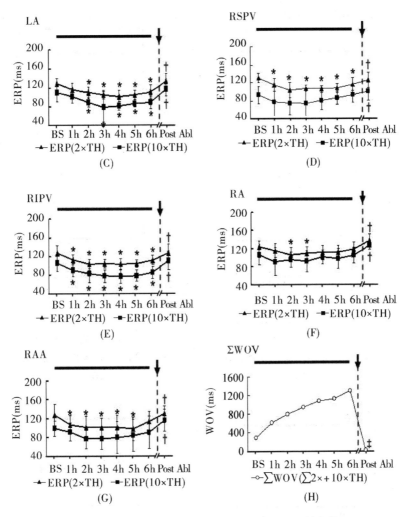

图 4-2 第 1 组中，GP 消融前后 ERP 和 WOV 的变化

消融前，在快速起搏的前 2 个小时，2×TH 和 10×TH ERP 显著缩短，更长时间的起搏不能进一步缩短 ERP。$\sum$ WOV 随着起搏时间延长而逐渐增加。GP 消融后，ERP 显著延长至起搏前水平，在所有部位均不能诱发房颤（$\sum$ WOV = 0）。

∗：与起搏前相比 $P<0.05$；†和‡：与消融前相比，$P<0.05$。

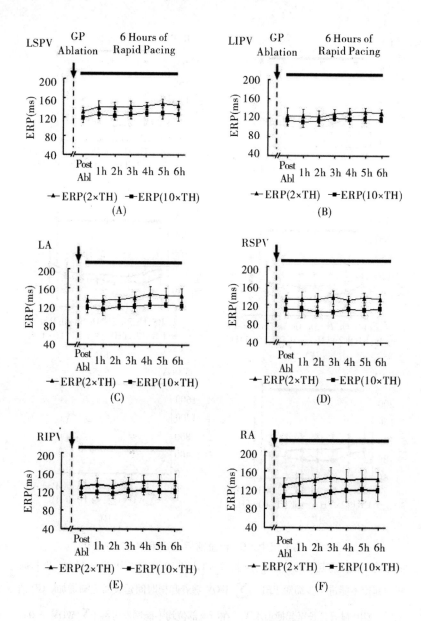

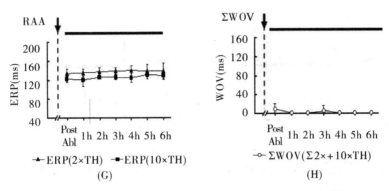

图4-3 第2组中，GP消融后，6h快速起搏不能缩短ERP和增加WOV
7条犬中的6条未能诱发AF，另一条犬在第3h(10×TH)诱发房颤，但
ΣWOV仅为10ms，而在第4~6h未能诱发AF。

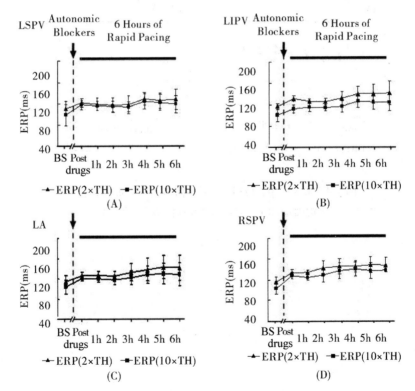

图4-4 第3组中，应用自主神经阻滞剂后，6h心耳起搏
不能缩短ERP，并且不能在任何部位诱发房颤

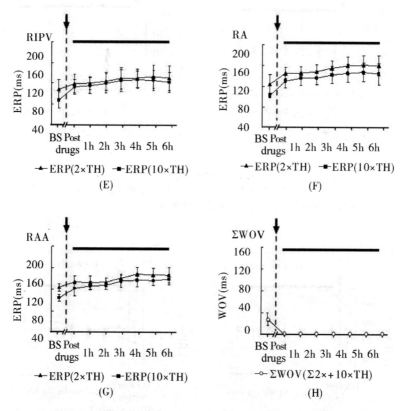

图4-4 第3组中，应用自主神经阻滞剂后，6h心耳起搏不能缩短ERP，并且不能在任何部位诱发房颤

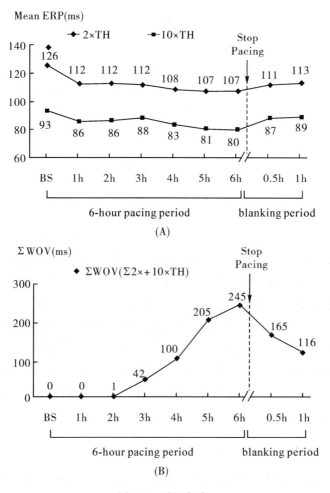

图 4-5 对照实验

快速心房起搏 6h 后,不消融 GP 而是给予 1h 的空白期,观察心房逆重构的程度。结果发现 ERP 即使在起搏中止后的 1h 内也没有显著变化,$\sum$ WOV 在起搏中止后的 1h 仍维持在 116ms。这说明,相对于 GP 定位和消融(<15min),心房逆重构是导致 GP 消融后 ERP 和 WOV 改变的次要因素。

第5章 综述：心房颤动的发生机制
——心脏内在自主神经系统的作用

鲁志兵　综　述
江　洪　审　校

心房颤动（房颤）是临床最常见的快速性心律失常，也是患者致残和致死的重要原因。尽管目前房颤的治疗领域已经取得了很大进展，但是房颤发生机制仍然存在较大争议。我们应该认识到：最佳的治疗方案应该建立在对机制的充分理解上。近年来，关于房颤发生机制的研究层出不穷，但是这些研究大多局限于肺静脉特殊的解剖特点和电生理性质，得出的结论也仅能解释房颤的某一个方面。本文总结房颤研究领域的主要研究成果，阐述房颤发生的可能机制，并重点介绍心脏内在自主神经系统在房颤发生和维持中的重要作用。

1. 阵发性房颤的发生机制

阵发性房颤主要由肺静脉肌袖内的局灶性快速电激动（Rapid Firing）引起[1]，产生 Firing 的机制从理论上有三种：自律性增高、微折返和触发活动。组织学研究发现，肺静脉内存在具有自律性的 P 细胞[2]，因此有学者认为由 P 细胞异常增加的自律性可能与肺静脉 Firing 有关[3]，但是下列现象并不支持这一推论：①P 细胞存在于肺静脉的远端，而 Firing 产生于肺静脉的近端；②舒张期除极是自律性电活动的特征性现象，然而有研究观察到 Firing 的起始并不存在舒张期除极[4]；③离体灌流的肺静脉肌袖并未观察到自发的电活动[5]，即使存在也非常微弱；④迷走神经兴奋抑制自律性但却有助于房颤的发生；⑤肺静脉电隔离术时，阻断肺静脉和心房之间的电连接从理论上不会影响肺静脉内的自律性，然而在绝大多数情况下 Firing 中止。

微折返被认为是 Firing 的另一个可能机制。Jalife[6]领导的研究小组在离体灌流的山羊心脏上观察到肺静脉-心房交界处的微折返可以产生 Firing 并驱动房颤，然而该模型是建立在高压力导致左心房扩大的基础上，类似于二尖瓣狭窄导致的房颤，可能并不能解释心脏结构正常的阵发性房颤。Po 等[4]观察到，在离体灌流的肺静脉口部可以诱发微折返，类似于临床观察到的 Firing。然而，微折返是在 Ach 存在的条件下，由早搏刺激诱发，微折返不会自发产生。在另外一项临床研究中，Patterson 等[7]用高密度篮状电极标测阵发性房颤起始后肺静脉内的电活动，结果发现微折返虽然存在，但是继发于局灶 Firing，并不是维持房颤所必需。以上研究并不能充分证明微折返在阵发性房颤中起到重要作用。

离体灌流的犬肺静脉-心房组织电生理研究结果表明[8,9]，由早后除极介导的触发活动可能是 Firing 的机制。由于肺静脉动作电位时程较短，在复极时其细胞内钙离子浓度仍然保持在较高水平，这给早后除极(EAD)的产生创造了良好的条件。肺静脉起源的 Firing 可被海豚毒素、阿托品或者阿替洛尔抑制，表明迷走成分和交感成分均参与了触发性 Firing 的产生。迷走兴奋导致肺静脉肌袖不应期进一步缩短，而交感兴奋则通过提升细胞内的钙离子浓度增加早后除极，Firing 在二者的共同作用下产生。为了验证这一推测，Patterson 等[8,9]在灌流的肺静脉组织中加入低浓度的 Ach 和 NE，结果诱发了高频 Firing。光学标测结果进一步支持触发活动是诱发 Firing 的机制[4]。最新的研究认为[10-12]，自主神经节(GP)可能是肺静脉 Firing 的幕后操纵者。GP 内含有大量迷走成分和部分交感成分[13]。当 GP 兴奋时，在迷走和交感的协同作用下，能在肺静脉内产生驱动房颤所需要的 Firing；GP 消融后，肺静脉内这种高频、紊乱的电活动消失，房颤难以诱发。从解剖学上看，每一根肺静脉均靠近相应的 GP，当 GP 兴奋时，在高浓度自主神经递质的作用下，肺静脉总是成为触发和驱动房颤最活跃的因素。有研究提示来自肺静脉以外(例如上腔静脉和Mashall韧带)的Firing，也与临近的GP有关[14]。以上研究似乎提示，GP才是阵发性房颤发生的关键因素，肺静脉起源的Firing只是GP兴奋的外在表现。

2. 慢性房颤的发生机制

目前的观点认为，多发子波折返是持续性或永久性房颤的主要维持机制。1995年，Wijffels等[15]发现对山羊的心房进行慢性快速起搏可以导致心房电重构。心房起搏时间越长，AF持续时间也越长，这种现象被称为"房颤致房颤"。房颤致房颤现象常常被用来模拟慢性房颤的发生机制。然而，在经典的"房颤致房颤"的动物模型中，Morillo等[16]报道了左房后壁临近肺静脉-心房交界区存在持续快速电激动，很可能是驱动房颤的关键因素。在类似的动物模型中，Zhou等[17]和Chou等[18]应用高精度光学标测方法观察到来自肺静脉的Firing与房颤的维持相关。这些研究说明，多发子波折返和局灶驱动同时参与了"房颤致房颤"的发生机制。我们最近的研究发现[19]，以GP为核心的心脏内在自主神经系统至少在"房颤致房颤"的急性期发挥了重要作用。在快速起搏6小时造成的急性心房电重构模型中，GP消融可以逆转和阻止心房电重构的发生，这说明心脏内在自主神经系统的激活本身可能是导致急性电重构的一个重要原因。需要引起重视的是该研究采用的是经典的"房颤致房颤"模型，这提示GP不仅仅跟"迷走性房颤"有关，而且参与了大多数房颤的发生机制。

3. 心-心反射(Cardio-Cardiac Reflex)与房颤

心脏内在自主神经系统主要由心包内大血管旁和心外膜的自主神经成分组成。心房表面的自主神经元聚集在肺静脉根部附近组成神经节(即GP)并被脂肪垫所包裹。GP内的自主神经元发出树突和轴突伸向临近的肺静脉、心房和远端的心耳。

目前我们对GP的作用所知甚少。传统观点认为[12,20]，心脏表面的GP不过是中枢神经系统通向心脏的中继站。然而，我们研究发现，GP不仅仅是上传下达的中继站，它还是心脏局部神经反射网络中的核心。当心脏局部的自主神经末梢兴奋时，刺激信号经传入纤维(afferent)激活GP，GP兴奋后又通过传出纤维(efferent)释放大量的神经递质(ACH和NE)到邻近的肺静脉、心房和远端的心耳，后三者再将兴奋信号源源不断地传回GP，这种快速的神经传导最终导致GP充分激活，临近的肺静脉在GP的驱使下总是成为触发和驱动房颤最活跃的因素。如上所述，心脏局部神经兴奋能在短时间内通过快速的神经传导使GP充分激活，我们称这种神经传导模式为心-心反射(Cardio-Cardiac Reflex，图5-1)。

我们通过一系列的实验研究发现心-心反射在心房颤动的发生和维持机制中起着重要的作用。当心脏局部自主神经末梢兴奋时，能通过心-心反射使临近的GP乃至整个心脏内在自主神经网络激活并释放大量自主神经递质至临近的肺静脉，在ACH和NE的协同作用下，肺静脉产生Firing，诱发和驱动房颤。当GP兴奋时，除了肺静脉产生Firing外，GP周围心房肌亦能产生紊乱、低频的电活动，类似临床观察到的碎裂电位(CFAE)。因此，CFAE可能也是GP兴奋的外在表现之一，也与心-心反射有关[12]。

4. 房颤的射频消融治疗

房颤的射频消融治疗是房颤治疗领域的重要进展[21,22]。大量临床研究已经证明了肺静脉电隔离对大部分房颤有效，但部分患者需要进行2~3次手术，因而肺静脉狭窄的风险增加。尽管肺静脉电隔离术已显示其有效性，但是这种术式需要隔离所有肺静脉，并不针对Firing的发生机制。已有多项临床研究表明，肺静脉电隔离并不是治愈房颤所必需[23,24]。某些消融术式并不要求达到肺静脉-心房双向阻滞但仍然能根治房颤。近年来，Cleveland电生理中心倡导的CFAE消融据报道能取得较高的成功率[25]，但从其公布的消融靶点图来看，CFAE所在区域包含了心房主要的GP(图5-2)[26,27]。这种术式的问题在于，由于CFAE电位在心房的分布广泛并且不稳定，因此消融过程中会不可避免地损伤无辜的心房肌，可能影响术后心房功能的恢复。最近发表的几个临床研究并未显示这种术式优于肺静脉隔离术[28,29]。

目前，尽管经严格设计的以 GP 消融为独立术式的导管消融报道尚未出现，但已有研究初步显示 GP 消融的有效性。Poppone 等[30]报道，环肺静脉消融时出现迷走反射而术后不能再诱发（即去迷走神经支配）的 101 例患者，在术后平均 12 个月的随访中，几乎所有患者房颤不再复发(99%，100/101)。Jackman 实验室的消融资料[31]也表明 GP 消融能显著提高肺静脉隔离的成功率。另一项临床研究表明[32]，即使放电消融时未出现明显的迷走反射，环肺静脉消融仍然能使 88% 迷走反射阳性位点（即 GP 所在位置）去神经支配，提示环肺静脉消融径线已经包含了大部分 GP 所在区域，环肺静脉消融所获得的成功率可能跟无意识地损伤 GP 有一定关系。外科微创消融资料[33]进一步支持 GP 在房颤中的重要作用：GP 消融后，在 6 个月的随访中，93%(14/15)的患者房颤消失。然而并不是所有研究都肯定 GP 消融的效果。Danik 等[34]最近发表的临床研究提示，GP 消融后房颤仍然能够被频率 20~50 Hz，电压 20~100 V 的高频刺激所诱发，但如此高强度的电刺激显然不适于评价房颤复发的可能性。该研究并未对 GP 消融的患者效果进行随访，因此 GP 消融的实际效果并不清楚。另有两项单纯从解剖位置消融 GP 的临床研究，得出的结论明显不同：Pokushalov 等[35]报道的 58 例房颤患者中（其中慢性房颤 21 例），GP 消融过程中有 94%(32/34)的患者房颤中止。在术后平均 7 个月的随访中，86%(50/58)的患者在无抗心律失常药物的情况下保持窦律。值得注意的是这些效果是在单次手术后取得的。然而 Kartitsis 等[36]报道的 19 例阵发性房颤患者，采用类似的 GP 消融后，大部分患者房颤复发，成功率显著低于环肺静脉消融术。这两个研究的共同问题在于，消融前没有采用高频电刺激验证 GP，消融后也没有检验 GP 是否被完全破坏，因此并不能算严格的"GP 消融"。Pokushalov 等在消融过程中，93%(54/58)的患者出现迷走反射，而 Kartitsis 等在消融过程中，仅 21%(4/19)的患者出现迷走反射，提示两个研究中 GP 被破坏的程度差异可能是导致结论不同的重要原因。毫无疑问，仅仅从解剖部位消融 GP 低估了完整的 GP 消融术式的成功率。

5. 结 论

现有的研究揭示了以 GP 为核心的心脏内在自主神经在房颤的发生和维持机制中发挥了重要作用，可能为确定房颤消融治疗的最佳靶点和制定最佳消融策略提供理论和实验依据。尽管已有的报道初步提示 GP 消融的有效性，但是我们期待经严格设计的以 GP 消融为独立术式的临床研究的出现。

参考文献

引言

[1] Haissaguerre M, Jais P, Shah DC, et al. Spontaneous initiation of atrial fibrillation by ectopic beats originating in the pulmonary veins. N Engl J Med. 1998, 339: 659-66.

[2] Nademanee K, McKenzie J, Kosar E, et al. A new approach for catheter ablation of atrial fibrillation: mapping of the electrophysiologic substrate. J Am Coll Cardiol. 2004, 43: 2044-53.

[3] Scherlag BJ, Nakagawa H, Jackman WM, et al. Electrical stimulation to identify neural elements on the heart: their role in atrial fibrillation. J Interv Card Electrophysiol. 2005, 13: 37-42.

[4] Chou CC, Nihei M, Zhou S, et al. Intracellular calcium dynamics and anisotropic reentry in isolated canine pulmonary veins and left atrium. Circulation. 2005, 111: 2889-97.

[5] Perez-Lugones A, McMahon JT, Ratliff NB, et al. Evidence of specialized conduction cells in human pulmonary veins of patients with atrial fibrillation. J Cardiovasc Electrophysiol. 2003, 14: 803-9.

[6] Chen YJ, Chen SA, Chang MS, et al. Arrhythmogenic activity of cardiac muscle in pulmonary veins of the dog: implication for the genesis of atrial fibrillation. Cardiovasc Res. 2000, 48: 265-73.

[7] Melnyk P, Ehrlich JR, Pourrier M, et al. Comparison of ion channel distribution and expression in cardiomyocytes of canine pulmonary veins versus left atrium. Cardiovasc Res. 2005, 65: 104-

16.

[8] Ehrlich JR, Cha TJ, Zhang L, et al. Cellular electrophysiology of canine pulmonary vein cardiomyocytes: action potential and ionic current properties. J Physiol. 2003, 551: 801-13.

[9] Scherlag BJ, Yamanashi W, Patel U, et al. Autonomically induced conversion of pulmonary vein focal firing into atrial fibrillation. J Am Coll Cardiol. 2005, 45: 1878-86.

[10] Patterson E, Po SS, Scherlag BJ, et al. Triggered firing in pulmonary veins initiated by in vitro autonomic nerve stimulation. Heart Rhythm. 2005, 2: 624-31.

[11] Patterson E, Lazzara R, Szabo B, et al. Sodium-calcium exchange initiated by the Ca2 + transient: an arrhythmia trigger within pulmonary veins. J Am Coll Cardiol. 2006, 47: 1196-206.

[12] Po SS, Scherlag BJ, Yamanashi WS, et al. Experimental model for paroxysmal atrial fibrillation arising at the pulmonary vein-atrial junctions. Heart Rhythm. 2006, 3: 201-8.

第1章

[1] Haissaguerre M, Jais P, Shah DC, et al. Spontaneous initiation of atrial fibrillation by ectopic beats originating in the pulmonary veins. N Engl J Med. 1998, 339: 659-66.

[2] Oral H, Knight BP, Tada H, et al. Pulmonary vein isolation for paroxysmal and persistent atrial fibrillation. Circulation. 2002, 105: 1077-81.

[3] Oral H, Pappone C, Chugh A, et al. Circumferential pulmonary-vein ablation for chronic atrial fibrillation. N Engl J Med. 2006, 354: 934-41.

[4] Chou CC, Nihei M, Zhou S, et al. Intracellular calcium dynamics and anisotropic reentry in isolated canine pulmonary veins and left atrium. Circulation. 2005, 111: 2889-97.

[5] Perez-Lugones A, McMahon JT, Ratliff NB, et al. Evidence of specialized conduction cells in human pulmonary veins of patients with atrial fibrillation. J Cardiovasc Electrophysiol. 2003, 14: 803-9.

[6] Chen YJ, Chen SA, Chang MS, et al. Arrhythmogenic activity of cardiac muscle in pulmonary veins of the dog: implication for the genesis of atrial fibrillation. Cardiovasc Res. 2000, 48: 265-73.

[7] Ehrlich JR, Cha TJ, Zhang L, et al. Cellular electrophysiology of canine pulmonary vein cardiomyocytes: action potential and ionic current properties. J Physiol. 2003, 551: 801-13.

[8] Patterson E, Po SS, Scherlag BJ, et al. Triggered firing in pulmonary veins initiated by in vitro autonomic nerve stimulation. Heart Rhythm. 2005, 2: 624-31.

[9] Patterson E, Lazzara R, Szabo B, et al. Sodium-calcium exchange initiated by the Ca2 + transient: an arrhythmia trigger within pulmonary veins. J Am Coll Cardiol. 2006, 47: 1196-206.

[10] Po SS, Scherlag BJ, Yamanashi WS, et al. Experimental model for paroxysmal atrial fibrillation arising at the pulmonary vein-atrial junctions. Heart Rhythm. 2006, 3: 201-8.

[11] Lu Z, Scherlag BJ, Lin J, et al. Autonomic mechanism for complex fractionated atrial electrograms: evidence by fast fourier transform analysis. J Cardiovasc Electrophysiol. 2008, 19: 835-42.

[12] Po SS, Li Y, Tang D, et al. Rapid and stable re-entry within the pulmonary vein as a mechanism initiating paroxysmal atrial fibrillation. J Am Coll Cardiol. 2005, 45: 1871-7.

[13] Yuan BX, Ardell JL, Hopkins DA, et al. Gross and microscopic anatomy of the canine intrinsic cardiac nervous system. Anat Rec. 1994, 239: 75-87.

[14] Pauza DH, Skripka V, Pauziene N. Morphology of the intrinsic cardiac nervous system in the dog: a whole-mount study employing histochemical staining with acetylcholinesterase. Cells Tissues Or-

gans. 2002, 172: 297-320.

[15] Makino M, Inoue S, Matsuyama TA, et al. Diverse myocardial extension and autonomic innervation on ligament of Marshall in humans. J Cardiovasc Electrophysiol. 2006, 17: 594-9.

[16] Ulphani JS, Arora R, Cain JH, et al. The ligament of Marshall as a parasympathetic conduit. Am J Physiol Heart Circ Physiol. 2007, 293: H1629-35.

[17] Doshi RN, Wu TJ, Yashima M, et al. Relation between ligament of Marshall and adrenergic atrial tachyarrhythmia. Circulation. 1999, 100: 876-83.

[18] Lin J, Scherlag BJ, Lu Z, et al. Inducibility of atrial and ventricular arrhythmias along the ligament of Marshall: Role of autonomic factors. J Cardiovasc Electrophysiol. 2008, 19: 955-62.

[19] Hou Y, Scherlag BJ, Lin J, et al. Ganglionated plexi modulate extrinsic cardiac autonomic nerve input: effects on sinus rate, atrioventricular conduction, refractoriness, and inducibility of atrial fibrillation. J Am Coll Cardiol. 2007, 50: 61-8.

[20] Armour JA. The little brain on the heart. Cleve Clin J Med. 2007, 74: S48-51.

[21] Schauerte P, Scherlag BJ, Patterson E, et al. Focal atrial fibrillation: experimental evidence for a pathophysiologic role of the autonomic nervous system. J Cardiovasc Electrophysiol. 2001, 12: 592-9.

[22] Lu Z, Scherlag BJ, Lin J, et al. Atrial fibrillation begets atrial fibrillation: autonomic mechanism for atrial electrical remodeling induced by short-term rapid atrial pacing. Circ Arrhythmia Electrophysiol. 2008, 1: 184-92.

[23] Wang TM, Chiang CE, Sheu JR, et al. Homogenous distribution of fast response action potentials in canine pulmonary vein sleeves: a contradictory report. Int J Cardiol. 2003, 89: 187-95.

[24] Kalifa J, Jalife J, Zaitsev AV, et al. Intra-atrial pressure increa-

ses rate and organization of waves emanating from the superior pulmonary veins during atrial fibrillation. Circulation. 2003, 108: 668-71.

[25] Patterson E, Jackman WM, Beckman KJ, et al. Spontaneous pulmonary vein firing in man: relationship to tachycardia-pause early afterdepolarizations and triggered arrhythmia in canine pulmonary veins in vitro. J Cardiovasc Electrophysiol. 2007, 18: 1067-75.

[26] Tan AY, Li H, Wachsmann-Hogiu S, et al. Autonomic innervation and segmental muscular disconnections at the human pulmonary vein-atrial junction: implications for catheter ablation of atrial-pulmonary vein junction. J Am Coll Cardiol. 2006, 48: 132-43.

[27] Zhang Y, Nakagawa H, Po SS, et al. Autonomic Ganglionated Plexi Stimulation Induces Fractionated Atrial Potentials in Contralateral Pulmonary Veins in Patients With Atrial Fibrillation. Circulation, 2006, 114: II_ 454 (abstra).

[28] Lemery R, Birnie D, Tang AS, et al. Feasibility study of endocardial mapping of ganglionated plexuses during catheter ablation of atrial fibrillation. Heart Rhythm. 2006, 3: 387-96.

第2章

[1] Tsai CF, Tai CT, Hsieh MH, et al. Initiation of atrial fibrillation by ectopic beats originating from the superior vena cava: electrophysiological characteristics and results of radiofrequency ablation. Circulation. 2000, 102: 67-74.

[2] Goya M, Ouyang F, Ernst S, et al. Electroanatomic mapping and catheter ablation of breakthroughs from the right atrium to the superior vena cava in patients with atrial fibrillation. Circulation. 2002, 106: 1317-20.

[3] Cooper TB, Hageman GR, James TN, et al. Neural effects on si-

nus rate and atrioventricular conduction produced by electrical stimulation from a transvenous electrode catheter in the canine right pulmonary artery. Circ Res. 1980, 46: 48-57.

[4] Mick JD, Wurster RD, Duff M et al. Epicardial sites for vagal mediation of sinoatrial function. Am J Physiol. 1992, 262: H1401-6.

[5] Chiou CW, Eble JN, Zipes DP. Efferent vagal innervation of the canine atria and sinus and atrioventricular nodes. The third fat pad. Circulation. 1997, 95: 2573-84.

[6] Patterson E, Po SS, Scherlag BJ, et al. Triggered firing in pulmonary veins initiated by in vitro autonomic nerve stimulation. Heart Rhythm. 2005, 2: 624-31.

[7] Patterson E, Lazzara R, Szabo B, et al. Sodium-calcium exchange initiated by the Ca2 + transient: an arrhythmia trigger within pulmonary veins. J Am Coll Cardiol. 2006, 47: 1196-206.

[8] Po SS, Scherlag BJ, Yamanashi WS, et al. Experimental model for paroxysmal atrial fibrillation arising at the pulmonary vein-atrial junctions. Heart Rhythm. 2006, 3: 201-8.

[9] Lu Z, Scherlag BJ, Lin J, et al. Autonomic mechanism for complex fractionated atrial electrograms: evidence by fast fourier transform analysis. J Cardiovasc Electrophysiol. 2008, 19: 835-42.

[10] Po SS, Li Y, Tang D, et al. Rapid and stable re-entry within the pulmonary vein as a mechanism initiating paroxysmal atrial fibrillation. J Am Coll Cardiol. 2005, 45: 1871-7.

[11] Lu Z, Scherlag BJ, Lin J, et al. Atrial fibrillation begets atrial fibrillation: autonomic mechanism for atrial electrical remodeling induced by short-term rapid atrial pacing. Circ Arrhythmia Electrophysiol. 2008, 1: 184-192.

[12] Lin J, Scherlag BJ, Lu Z, et al. Inducibility of atrial and ventricular arrhythmias along the ligament of Marshall: Role of autonomic factors. J Cardiovasc Electrophysiol. 2008, 19: 955-62.

[13] Schauerte P, Scherlag BJ, Patterson E, et al. Focal atrial fibrillation: experimental evidence for a pathophysiologic role of the autonomic nervous system. J Cardiovasc Electrophysiol. 2001, 12: 592-9.

[14] Pauza DH, Skripka V, Pauziene N. Morphology of the intrinsic cardiac nervous system in the dog: a whole-mount study employing histochemical staining with acetylcholinesterase. Cells Tissues Organs. 2002, 172: 297-320.

[15] Pauza DH, Skripka V, Pauziene N, et al. Anatomical study of the neural ganglionated plexus in the canine right atrium: implications for selective denervation and electrophysiology of the sinoatrial node in dog. Anat Rec. 1999, 255: 271-94.

[16] Horackova M, Armour JA, Byczko Z. Distribution of intrinsic cardiac neurons in whole-mount guinea pig atria identified by multiple neurochemical coding. A confocal microscope study. Cell Tissue Res. 1999, 297: 409-21.

[17] Arruda M, Mlcochova H, Prasad SK, et al. Electrical Isolation of the Superior Vena Cava: An Adjunctive Strategy to Pulmonary Vein Antrum Isolation Improving the Outcome of AF Ablation. J Cardiovasc Electrophysiol. 2007, 18: 1261-6.

[18] Tsai CF, Tai CT, Hsieh MH, et al. Initiation of atrial fibrillation by ectopic beats originating from the superior vena cava: electrophysiological characteristics and results of radiofrequency ablation. Circulation. 2000, 102: 67-74.

第3章

[1] Nademanee K, McKenzie J, Kosar E, et al. A new approach for catheter ablation of atrial fibrillation: Mapping of the electrophysiologic substrate. J Am Coll Cardiol. 2004, 43: 2044-53.

[2] Oral H, Chugh A, Good E, et al. Radiofrequency catheter ablation of chronic atrial fibrillation guided by complex electrograms.

Circulation. 2007, 115: 2606-12.

[3] Gardner PI, Ursell PC, Fenoglio JJ Jr, et al. Electrophysiologic and anatomic basis for fractionated electrograms recorded from healed myocardial infarcts. Circulation. 1985, 72: 596-611.

[4] Berenfeld O, Zaitsev AV, Mironov SF, et al. Frequency-dependent breakdown of wave propagation into fibrillatory conduction across the pectinate muscle network in the isolated sheep right atrium. Circ Res. 2002, 90: 1173-80

[5] Mansour M, Mandapati R, Berenfeld O, et al. Left-to-right gradient of atrial frequencies during acute atrial fibrillation in the isolated sheep heart. Circulation. 2001, 103: 2631-6.

[6] Jalife J, Berenfeld O, Mansour M. Mother rotors and fibrillatory conduction: a mechanism of atrial fibrillation. Cardiovasc Res. 2002, 54: 204-6.

[7] Oral H, Chugh A, Yoshida K, et al. A randomized assessment of the incremental role of ablation of complex fractionated atrial electrograms after antral pulmonary vein isolation for long-lasting persistent atrial fibrillation. J Am Coll Cardiol. 2009, 53: 782-9.

[8] Deisenhofer I, Estner H, Reents T, et al. Does Electrogram Guided Substrate Ablation Add to the Success of Pulmonary Vein Isolation in Patients with Paroxysmal Atrial Fibrillation? A Prospective, Randomized Study. J Cardiovasc Electrophysiol. Doi: 10.1111/j.1540-8167. 2008. 01379. x

[9] Estner HL, Hessling G, Ndrepepa G, et al. Electrogram-guided substrate ablation with or without pulmonary vein isolation in patients with persistent atrial fibrillation. Europace. 2008, 10: 1281-7.

[10] Oketani N, Lockwood E, Nademanee K. Incidence and mode of A. F. termination during substrate ablation of A. F. guided solely by complex fractionated atrial electrogram mapping, Circulation. 2008, 118: S925. (abstr)

[11] Verma A, Patel D, Famey T, et al, Efficacy of adjuvant anterior

left atrial ablation during intracardiac echocardiography-guided pulmonary vein antrum isolation for atrial fibrillation. J Cardiovasc Electrophysiol. 2007, 18: 151-6.

[12] Nakagawa H, Jackman WM, Scherlag BJ, et al. Relationship of complex fractionated atrial electrograms during atrial fibrillation to the location of cardiac autonomic ganglionated plexi in patients with atrial fibrillation. Circulation. 2005, 112: II-746. (Abstr)

[13] Katritsis D, Giazitzoglou E, Sougiannis D, et al. Complex fractionated atrial electrograms at anatomic sites of ganglionated plexi in atrial fibrillation. Europace. 2009, 11: 308-15.

[14] Po SS, Scherlag BJ, Yamanashi WS, et al. Experimental model for paroxysmal atrial fibrillation arising at the pulmonary vein-atrial junctions. Heart Rhythm. 2006, 3: 201-8.

[15] Kalifa J, Tanaka K, Zaitsev AV, et al. Mechanisms of wave fractionation at boundaries of high-frequency excitation in the posterior left atrium of the isolated sheep heart during atrial fibrillation. Circulation. 2006, 113: 626-33.

[16] Lin J, Scherlag BJ, Zhou J, et al. Autonomic mechanism to explain complex fractionated atrial electrograms (CFAE). J Cardiovasc Electrophysiol. 2007, 18: 1197-205.

[17] Zhou J, Scherlag BJ, Edwards J, et al. Gradients of Atrial Refractoriness and Inducibility of Atrial Fibrillation due to Stimulation of Ganglionated Plexi. J Cardiovasc Electrophysiol. 2007, 18: 83-90.

[18] Yuan BX, Ardell JL, Hopkins DA, et al. Gross and microscopic anatomy of the canine intrinsic cardiac nervous system. Anat Rec. 1994, 239: 75-87.

[19] Chevalier P, Tabib A, Meyronnet D, et al. Quantitative study of nerves of the human left atrium. Heart Rhythm. 2005, 2: 518-22.

[20] Randall WC, Milosavljevic M, Wurster RD, et al. Selective va-

gal innervation of the heart. Ann Clin Lab Sci. 1986, 16: 198-208.

[21] Pauza DH, Skripka V, Pauziene N. Morphology of the intrinsic cardiac nervous system in the dog: a whole-mount study employing histochemical staining with acetylcholinesterase. Cells Tissues Organs. 2002, 172: 297-320.

[22] Armour JA. The little brain on the heart. Cleve Clin J Med. 2007, 74: S48-51.

[23] Rostock T, Rotter M, Sanders P, et al. High-density activation mapping of fractionated electrograms in the atria of patients with paroxysmal atrial fibrillation. Heart Rhythm. 2006, 3: 27-34.

[24] Lancaster R. Measurement of the rate of acetylcholine diffusion through a brain slice and its significance in studies of the cellular distribution of acetylcholinesterase. J Neurochem. 1971, 18: 2329-34.

第4章

[1] Wijffels MC, Kirchhof CJ, Dorland R, et al. Atrial fibrillation begets atrial fibrillation. A study in awake chronically instrumented goats. Circulation. 1995, 92: 1954-68.

[2] Yue L, Melnyk P, Gaspo R, et al. Molecular mechanisms underlying ionic remodeling in a dog model of atrial fibrillation. Circ Res. 1999, 84: 776-84.

[3] Bosch RF, Scherer CR, Rüb N, et al. Molecular mechanisms of early electrical remodeling: transcriptional downregulation of ion channel subunits reduces I(Ca, L) and I(to) in rapid atrial pacing in rabbits. J Am Coll Cardiol. 2003, 41: 858-69.

[4] Po SS, Scherlag BJ, Yamanashi WS, et al. Experimental model for paroxysmal atrial fibrillation arising at the pulmonary vein-atrial junctions. Heart Rhythm. 2006, 3: 201-8.

[5] Zhou J, Scherlag BJ, Edwards J, et al. Gradients of Atrial Re-

fractoriness and Inducibility of Atrial Fibrillation due to Stimulation of Ganglionated Plexi. J Cardiovasc Electrophysiol. 2007, 18: 83-90.

[6] Patterson E, Po SS, Scherlag BJ, et al. Triggered firing in pulmonary veins initiated by in vitro autonomic nerve stimulation. Heart Rhythm. 2005, 2: 624-31.

[7] Po SS, Li Y, Tang D, et al. Rapid and stable re-entry within the pulmonary vein as a mechanism initiating paroxysmal atrial fibrillation. J Am Coll Cardiol. 2005, 45: 1871-7.

[8] Scherlag BJ, Nakagawa H, Jackman WM, et al. Electrical stimulation to identify neural elements on the heart: their role in atrial fibrillation. J Interv Card Electrophysiol. 2005, 13: 37-42.

[9] Hou Y, Scherlag BJ, Lin J, et al. Interactive atrial neural network: Determining the connections between ganglionated plexi. Heart Rhythm. 2007, 4: 56-63.

[10] Hou Y, Scherlag BJ, Lin J, et al. Ganglionated plexi modulate extrinsic cardiac autonomic nerve input: effects on sinus rate, atrioventricular conduction, refractoriness, and inducibility of atrial fibrillation. J Am Coll Cardiol. 2007, 50: 61-8.

[11] Lin J, Scherlag BJ, Zhou J, et al. Autonomic mechanism to explain complex fractionated atrial electrograms (CFAE). J Cardiovasc Electrophysiol. 2007, 18: 1197-205.

[12] Lee KW, Everett TH 4th, Rahmutula D, et al. Pirfenidone prevents the development of a vulnerable substrate for atrial fibrillation in a canine model of heart failure. Circulation. 2006, 114: 1703-12.

[13] Wijffels MC, Kirchhof CJ, Dorland R, et al Electrical remodeling due to atrial fibrillation in chronically instrumented conscious goats: roles of neurohumoral changes, ischemia, atrial stretch, and high rate of electrical activation. Circulation. 1997, 96: 3710-20.

[14] Moe GK, Abildskov JA. Atrial fibrillation as a self-sustaining arrhythmia independent of focal discharge. Am Heart J. 1959, 58: 59-70.

[15] Haissaguerre M, Jais P, Shah DC, et al. Spontaneous initiation of atrial fibrillation by ectopic beats originating in the pulmonary veins. N Engl J Med. 1998, 339: 659-66.

[16] Patterson E, Jackman WM, Beckman KJ, et al. Spontaneous Pulmonary Vein Firing in Man: Relationship to Tachycardia-Pause Early Afterdepolarizations and Triggered Arrhythmia in Canine Pulmonary Veins In Vitro. J Cardiovasc Electrophysiol. 2007, 18: 1067-75

[17] Morillo CA, Klein GJ, Jones DL, et al. Chronic rapid atrial pacing. Structural, functional, and electrophysiological characteristics of a new model of sustained atrial fibrillation. Circulation. 1995, 91: 1588-95.

[18] Zhou S, Chang CM, Wu TJ, et al. Nonreentrant focal activations in pulmonary veins in canine model of sustained atrial fibrillation. Am J Physiol Heart Circ Physiol. 2002, 283: H1244-52.

[19] Chou CC, Zhou S, Tan AY, et al. High-density mapping of pulmonary veins and left atrium during ibutilide administration in a canine model of sustained atrial fibrillation. Am J Physiol Heart Circ Physiol. 2005, 289: H2704-13.

[20] Tan AY, Li H, Wachsmann-Hogiu S, et al. Autonomic innervation and segmental muscular disconnections at the human pulmonary vein-atrial junction: implications for catheter ablation of atrial-pulmonary vein junction. J Am Coll Cardiol. 2006, 48: 132-43.

[21] Neuberger HR, Schotten U, Blaauw Y, et al. Chronic atrial dilation, electrical remodeling, and atrial fibrillation in the goat. J Am Coll Cardiol. 2006, 47: 644-53.

[22] Yamashita T, Murakawa Y, Hayami N, et al. Short-term effects

of rapid pacing on mRNA level of voltage-dependent K(+) channels in rat atrium: electrical remodeling in paroxysmal atrial tachycardia. Circulation. 2000, 101: 2007-14.

[23] Cha TJ, Ehrlich JR, Chartier D, et al. Kir3-based inward rectifier potassium current: potential role in atrial tachycardia remodeling effects on atrial repolarization and arrhythmias. Circulation. 2006, 113: 1730-7.

[24] Jayachandran JV, Sih HJ, Winkle W, et al. Atrial fibrillation produced by prolonged rapid atrial pacing is associated with heterogeneous changes in atrial sympathetic innervation. Circulation. 2000, 101: 1185-91.

[25] Cha TJ, Ehrlich JR, Chartier D, et al. Kir3-based inward rectifier potassium current: potential role in atrial tachycardia remodeling effects on atrial repolarization and arrhythmias. Circulation. 2006, 113: 1730-7.

[26] Yeh YH, Qi X, Shiroshita-Takeshita A, et al. Atrial tachycardia induces remodelling of muscarinic receptors and their coupled potassium currents in canine left atrial and pulmonary vein cardiomyocytes. Br J Pharmacol. 2007, 152: 1021-32.

第5章

[1] Haissaguerre M, Jais P, Shah DC, et al. Spontaneous initiation of atrial fibrillation by ectopic beats originating in the pulmonary veins. N Engl J Med. 1998, 339: 659-66.

[2] Perez-Lugones A, McMahon JT, Ratliff NB, et al. Evidence of specialized conduction cells in human pulmonary veins of patients with atrial fibrillation. J Cardiovasc Electrophysiol. 2003, 14: 803-9.

[3] Chen YJ, Chen SA, Chang MS, et al. Arrhythmogenic activity of cardiac muscle in pulmonary veins of the dog: implication for the genesis of atrial fibrillation. Cardiovasc Res. 2000, 48: 265-73.

[4] Po SS, Li Y, Tang D, et al. Rapid and stable re-entry within the pulmonary vein as a mechanism initiating paroxysmal atrial fibrillation. J Am Coll Cardiol. 2005, 45: 1871-7.

[5] Wang TM, Chiang CE, Sheu JR, et al. Homogenous distribution of fast response action potentials in canine pulmonary vein sleeves: a contradictory report. Int J Cardiol. 2003, 89: 187-95.

[6] Kalifa J, Jalife J, Zaitsev AV, et al. Intra-atrial pressure increases rate and organization of waves emanating from the superior pulmonary veins during atrial fibrillation. Circulation. 2003, 108: 668-71.

[7] Patterson E, Jackman WM, Beckman KJ, et al. Spontaneous pulmonary vein firing in man: relationship to tachycardia-pause early afterdepolarizations and triggered arrhythmia in canine pulmonary veins in vitro. J Cardiovasc Electrophysiol. 2007, 18: 1067-75.

[8] Patterson E, Po SS, Scherlag BJ, et al. Triggered firing in pulmonary veins initiated by in vitro autonomic nerve stimulation. Heart Rhythm. 2005, 2: 624-31.

[9] Patterson E, Lazzara R, Szabo B, et al. Sodium-calcium exchange initiated by the Ca2 + transient: an arrhythmia trigger within pulmonary veins. J Am Coll Cardiol. 2006, 47: 1196-206.

[10] Po SS, Scherlag BJ, Yamanashi WS, et al. Experimental model for paroxysmal atrial fibrillation arising at the pulmonary vein-atrial junctions. Heart Rhythm. 2006, 3: 201-8.

[11] Scherlag BJ, Hou YL, Lin J, et al. An acute model for atrial fibrillation arising from a peripheral atrial site: evidence for primary and secondary triggers. J Cardiovasc Electrophysiol. 2008, 19: 519-27.

[12] Lu Z, Scherlag BJ, Lin J, et al. Autonomic mechanism for complex fractionated atrial electrograms: evidence by fast fourier transform analysis. J Cardiovasc Electrophysiol. 2008, 19: 835-42.

[13] Tan AY, Li H, Wachsmann-Hogiu S, et al. Autonomic innerva-

tion and segmental muscular disconnections at the human pulmonary vein-atrial junction: implications for catheter ablation of atrial-pulmonary vein junction. J Am Coll Cardiol. 2006, 48: 132-43.

[14] Lin J, Scherlag BJ, Lu Z, et al. Inducibility of atrial and ventricular arrhythmias along the ligament of Marshall: Role of autonomic factors. J Cardiovasc Electrophysiol. 2008, 19: 955-62.

[15] Wijffels MC, Kirchhof CJ, Dorland R, et al. Atrial fibrillation begets atrial fibrillation. A study in awake chronically instrumented goats. Circulation. 1995, 92: 1954-68.

[16] Morillo CA, Klein GJ, Jones DL, et al. Chronic rapid atrial pacing. Structural, functional, and electrophysiological characteristics of a new model of sustained atrial fibrillation. Circulation. 1995, 91: 1588-95.

[17] Zhou S, Chang CM, Wu TJ, et al. Nonreentrant focal activations in pulmonary veins in canine model of sustained atrial fibrillation. Am J Physiol Heart Circ Physiol. 2002, 283: H1244-52.

[18] Chou CC, Zhou S, Tan AY, et al. High-density mapping of pulmonary veins and left atrium during ibutilide administration in a canine model of sustained atrial fibrillation. Am J Physiol Heart Circ Physiol. 2005, 289: H2704-13.

[19] Lu Z, Scherlag BJ, Lin J, et al. Atrial fibrillation begets atrial fibrillation: autonomic mechanism for atrial electrical remodeling induced by short-term rapid atrial pacing. Circ Arrhythmia Electrophysiol. 2008, 1: 184-192.

[20] Scherlag BJ, Hou YL, Lin J, et al. An acute model for atrial fibrillation arising from a peripheral atrial site: evidence for primary and secondary triggers. J Cardiovasc Electrophysiol. 2008, 19: 519-27.

[21] Oral H, Knight BP, Tada H, et al. Pulmonary vein isolation for paroxysmal and persistent atrial fibrillation.. Circulation. 2002,

105: 1077-81.

[22] Oral H, Pappone C, Chugh A, et al. Circumferential pulmonary-vein ablation for chronic atrial fibrillation.. N Engl J Med. 2006, 354: 934-41.

[23] Lemola K, Oral H, Chugh A, et al. Pulmonary vein isolation as an end point for left atrial circumferential ablation of atrial fibrillation. J Am Coll Cardiol. 2005, 46: 1060-1066.

[24] Stabile G, Turco P, La Rocca V, et al. Is pulmonary vein isolation necessary for curing atrial fibrillation? Circulation. 2003, 108: 657-60.

[25] Nademanee K, McKenzie J, Kosar E, et al. A new approach for catheter ablation of atrial fibrillation: Mapping of the electrophysiologic substrate. J Am Coll Cardiol. 2004, 43: 2044-53.

[26] Nakagawa H, Jackman WM, Scherlag BJ, et al. Relationship of complex fractionated atrial electrograms during atrial fibrillation to the location of cardiac autonomic ganglionated plexi in patients with atrial fibrillation (Abstract). Circulation. 2005, 112: II-746.

[27] Katritsis D, Giazitzoglou E, Sougiannis D, et al. Complex fractionated atrial electrograms at anatomic sites of ganglionated plexi in atrial fibrillation. Europace. 2009, 11: 308-15.

[28] Oral H, Chugh A, Yoshida K, et al. A randomized assessment of the incremental role of ablation of complex fractionated atrial electrograms after antral pulmonary vein isolation for long-lasting persistent atrial fibrillation. J Am Coll Cardiol. 2009, 53: 782-9.

[29] Deisenhofer I, Estner H, Reents T, et al. Does Electrogram Guided Substrate Ablation Add to the Success of Pulmonary Vein Isolation in Patients with Paroxysmal Atrial Fibrillation? A Prospective, Randomized Study. J Cardiovasc Electrophysiol. Doi. 10.1111/j. 1540-8167. 2008. 01379. x. [Epub ahead of print]

[30] Pappone C, Santinelli V, Manguso F, et al. Pulmonary vein

denervation enhances long-term benefit after circumferential ablation for paroxysmal atrial fibrillation. Circulation, 2004, 109: 327-34.

[31] Scherlag BJ, Nakagawa H, Jackman WM, et al. Electrical stimulation to identify neural elements on the heart: their role in atrial fibrillation. J Interv Card Electrophysiol, 2005, 13: 37-42.

[32] Lemery R, Birnie D, Tang AS, et al. Feasibility study of endocardial mapping of ganglionated plexuses during catheter ablation of atrial fibrillation. Heart Rhythm. 2006, 3: 387-96.

[33] Mehall JR, Kohut RM Jr, Schneeberger EW, et al. Intraoperative epicardial electrophysiologic mapping and isolation of autonomic ganglionic plexi. Ann Thorac Surg, 2007, 83: 538-41.

[34] Danik S, Neuzil P, d'Avila A, et al. Evaluation of catheter ablation of periatrial ganglionic plexi in patients with atrial fibrillation. Am J Cardiol. 2008, 102: 578-83.

[35] Pokushalov E, Turov A, Shugayev P, et al. Catheter ablation of left atrial ganglionated plexi for atrial fibrillation. Asian Cardiovasc Thorac Ann. 2008, 16: 194-201.

[36] Katritsis D, Giazitzoglou E, Sougiannis D, et al. Anatomic approach for ganglionic plexi ablation in patients with paroxysmal atrial fibrillation. Am J Cardiol. 2008, 102: 330-4.

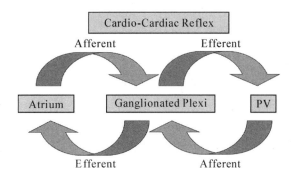

图 5-1　心-心反射(Cardio-Cardiac Reflex)示意图

心脏局部(PV 或 Atrium)的激动能通过传入纤维(afferent)激活神经节(ganglionated plexi，GP)，GP 兴奋后又通过传出纤维在外周释放大量自主神经递质，兴奋 GP 周边和远端结构。

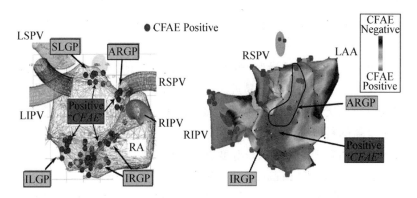

图 5-2　碎裂电位(CFAE)和自主神经节(GP)的分布
　　　　CFAE 分布区域包含了 GP 所在部位。

后　记

五年漫漫求学之路，在师长、亲友的多方支持下，走得辛苦却也收获满囊。

最感谢的是我的恩师江洪教授，他治学严谨，学识渊博，思想深邃，视野开阔，是我一生学习的榜样。五年来恩师不仅教会了我最前沿的科学知识和临床技能，还使我掌握了科学的思维方法，明白了许多为人处世的道理，为我今后独立思考问题、解决问题打下了坚实的基础。恩师严于律己、宽以待人的崇高风范，朴实无华、平易近人的人格魅力与无微不至、感人至深的关怀，令我如沐春风，倍感温馨。我将终生谨记恩师五年的教诲，以导师的指引作为前进的方向。

衷心感谢美国的导师 Sunny S. Po 教授，他渊博雄厚的学识、严谨认真的学术态度、平易近人的大师风范、宽厚仁慈的人格魅力以及对我如父般的关怀令我终生难忘。Po 教授的教导不仅使我掌握了全新的科研思路和严谨的临床思路，更是让我见识了世界最先进的导管消融理论和方法，让我在以后的工作和科研中打下了坚实的基础。衷心感谢 Benjamin J. Scherlag 教授、Warren M. Jackman 教授、Eugen Patterson 教授、Ralph Lazzara 教授，是你们让我有机会站在世界科学的最前沿，领略到这些科学伟人们的风采。衷心感谢侯应龙教授、林佳雄博士、牛国栋博士、余锂镭博士、李树岩教授和张媛教授对我实验上的支持和帮助。

衷心感谢武汉大学人民医院心内科全体老师对我工作、学习、科研和生活给予的无私帮助。衷心感谢心导管室黄鹤博士、王晓红老师、刘华芬老师、刘秀娟老师和杨新红老师多年来对我的关心、指导和培养。衷心感谢 211 实验室王腾老师、王兮老师和胡萍老师

后　记

等对我实验工作的悉心指导和支持。衷心感谢赵冬冬博士、朱丽华博士、胡笑容博士、温华知博士和何博博士等同学对我实验的大力帮助，几年来与他们并肩奋斗的同窗之谊将是我今生最宝贵的回忆。

感谢最亲爱的父母和爱人对我学业一贯的支持，对我生活无微不至的照顾。没有他们默默无闻的奉献，我不可能取得今天的成绩。他们的理解、支持和爱永远是我力量的源泉和前进的动力。

最后，再次向所有关心和帮助过我的老师、同学和亲人致以最诚挚的感谢！在我今后的人生道路上，我会继续努力，不辜负你们的期望！

武汉大学优秀博士学位论文文库

已出版：

- 基于双耳线索的移动音频编码研究／陈水仙　著
- 多帧影像超分辨率复原重建关键技术研究／谢伟　著
- Copula函数理论在多变量水文分析计算中的应用研究／陈璐　著
- 大型地下洞室群地震响应与结构面控制型围岩稳定研究／张雨霆　著
- 迷走神经诱发心房颤动的电生理和离子通道基础研究／赵庆彦　著
- 心房颤动的自主神经机制研究／鲁志兵　著
- 氧化应激状态下维持黑素小体蛋白低免疫原性的分子机制研究／刘小明　著
- 实流形在复流形中的全纯不变量／尹万科　著
- MITA介导的细胞抗病毒反应信号转导及其调节机制／钟波　著
- 图书馆数字资源选择标准研究／唐琼　著
- 年龄结构变动与经济增长：理论模型与政策建议／李魁　著
- 积极一般预防理论研究／陈金林　著
- 海洋石油开发环境污染法律救济机制研究／高翔　著
    ——以美国墨西哥湾漏油事故和我国渤海湾漏油事故为视角
- 中国共产党人政治忠诚观研究／徐霞　著
- 现代汉语属性名词语义特征研究／许艳平　著
- 论马克思的时间概念／熊进　著
- 晚明江南诗学研究／张清河　著